Sameh Achoura
Hajer Hammami

Tumors of the cranial vault

Sameh Achoura
Hajer Hammami

Tumors of the cranial vault

Support

ScienciaScripts

Cover image: www.ingimage.com

This book is a translation from the original published under ISBN 978-620-6-72070-6.

Publisher:
Sciencia Scripts
is a trademark of
Dodo Books Indian Ocean Ltd. and OmniScriptum S.R.L publishing group

120 High Road, East Finchley, London, N2 9ED, United Kingdom
Str. Armeneasca 28/1, office 1, Chisinau MD-2012, Republic of Moldova, Europe
Printed at: see last page
ISBN: 978-620-8-06038-1

CONTENTS

INTRODUCTION

Tumors of the skull vault are rare and very diverse, and are dominated in frequency by secondary lesions. They account for 0.8% to 2% of all bone tumors.

They are discovered either by chance, during a radiological work-up, or systematically during an extension work-up for certain haemopathies or osteophilic cancers.

The clinical picture is not very suggestive.

The neuroradiological workup relies mainly on CT scans.

Histological examination is necessary to define the histological type and grade of the tumor, which will subsequently determine the therapeutic attitude and prognosis.

Treatment is surgical, with chemotherapy and/or radiotherapy necessary in some cases. Sometimes, abstention is required.

Our study concerns a series of 20 cases of skull vault tumor, collected in the neurosurgery department of the Hôpital Militaire Principal d'Instruction in Tunis over a period of 17 years.

The objectives of this study are :

- Study the epidemiological, clinical, radiological and therapeutic aspects of cranial vault tumours;
- Assess short- and long-term evolution and prognosis;
- Compare our results with those in the literature.

PATIENTS AND METHODS

I. Patients

This is a retrospective analytical study of 20 observations of primary and secondary cranial vault tumors.

1. Inclusion criteria

We included patients followed and managed for vault tumor at the neurosurgery department of the main military hospital of instruction in Tunis, between 2000 and 2016.

2. Exclusion criteria

We have excluded :

- Patients diagnosed with tumors of the base extending to the cranial vault, meningiomas invading the cranial vault and infectious lesions.
- Age under 20.
- Patients lost to follow-up.

II. Study methods

1. Data collection

We collected and studied data on these patients from observation notebooks.

All of these data were compiled using a data entry form (Appendix 1) highlighting the clinical, radiological and anatomopathological characteristics:

- Patient identification ;
- The consultation period ;
- Discovery mode ;
- Examination of the swelling;
- Neurological examination;
- Somatic examination ;
- Radiological (Rx, CT, MRI) and biological data;
- The different treatment modalities: medical treatment, surgical treatment, radiotherapy, chemotherapy;
- Anatomopathological examination ;
- Short- and long-term trends ;

2. Data analysis and statistical study

It is a descriptive study of anamnestic, physical, radiological and evolutionary elements.

Data were entered using Excel and analyzed using SPSS version 21.0.

Quantitative variables were expressed as averages and percentages.

RESULTS

I. Overall results

A. Epidemiological data

1.age distribution

Our patients ranged in age from 20 to 75, with an average age of 47.4. 25% (5 patients) were under 35, and 20% (4 patients) were over 60.

Table IAge distribution of patients

Age	Number		%
	Benign	Malignant	
20 à 29	4		20
30 à 39	3		15
40 à 49	2	1	15
50 à 59	2	3	25
60 à 69	1	2	15
70 à 79		2	10
Total	12	8	

The figure below shows the age distribution of these lesions in our series:

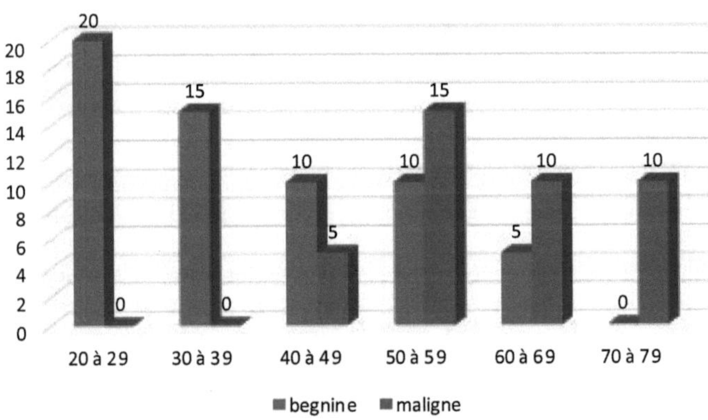

Figure 1Patient distribution by age

The distribution of lesions shows a frequency peak in the 6ème decade.

However, benign lesions predominated in the 3ème decade (20%), compared with 5% in the 7ème decade, while malignant lesions were more frequent in the 6ème decade (15%).

2. Breakdown by gender

The distribution of patients by gender revealed a slight male predominance, with an M/F sex ratio of 1.2.

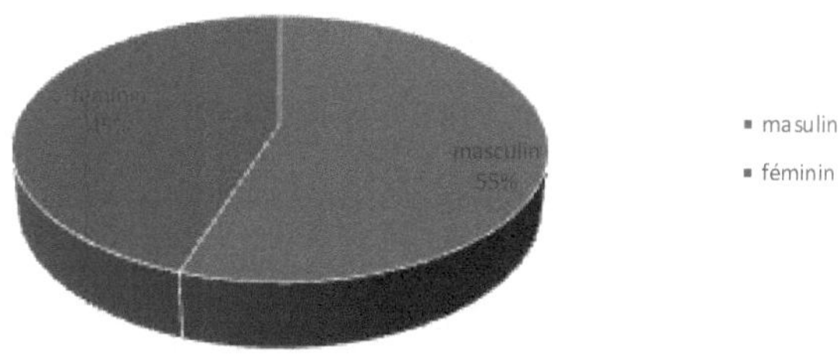

Figure 2Lesion distribution by gender

3. History

In the case of benign lesions, no general history was noted.

In addition, the notion of benign head trauma preceding the discovery of an arch lesion has been reported, with an average delay of 12 months and extremes ranging from 6 months to 10 years.

Three patients suffered head trauma, i.e. 15% of our series.

For secondary lesions, one patient was being monitored for dyslipidemia.

A patient was treated 10 years ago for common pulmonary tuberculosis.

A patient followed in the ophthalmology department for adenocarcinoma of the lacrimal gland.

A patient undergoing cataract surgery and total thyroidectomy.

B. Clinical data

1. functional signs

Cranial swelling was noted in 9 patients.

Headaches were present in 8 patients.

2.physical signs

Physical examination revealed :

Most of our patients are in good general condition.

One patient had an altered general condition with a karnofsky of 60% (WHO 3).

Swelling in 9 patients: soft in 2, firm in 4 and hard in 3.

Pain on palpation was reported in 4 patients.

The appearance of the skin opposite the lesion was mentioned in 9 patients: it was normal in 8 and inflammatory in only one case.

A patient was found to have a hard breast mass with a long axis of 4 cm.

Bronchial syndrome in one patient.

One patient had a hard, painless mass on rectal examination.

The clinical picture on admission consisted essentially of :

- Headaches: 8 patients (40%)

- Local swelling of the skull vault: 9 patients (45%)
- Incidental findings:3 patients (15%).

Neurological disorders were not observed in our patients.

Table II:Distribution of patients according to clinical signs

	Number of patients	Percentage
Headaches	8	40 %
Local swelling	9	45%
Neurological deficit	0	0%
A chance discovery	3	15%

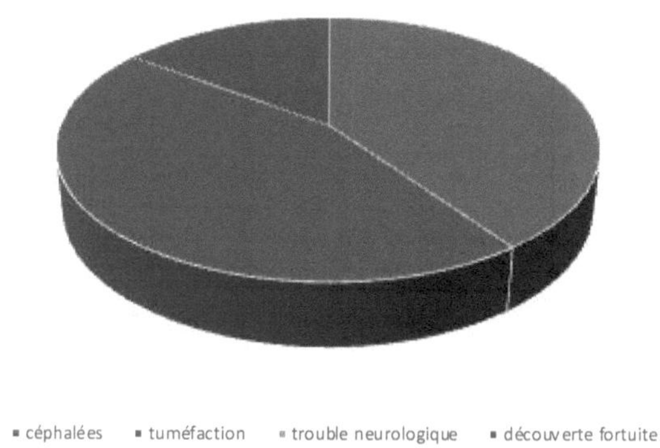

Figure 3Distribution of patients according to clinical signs

C. Paraclinical data

1. Skull X-ray

Seven patients had undergone standard radiographic explorations (frontal skull; profile).

X-rays of the skull showed bone lysis in 2 cases, osteocondensation in 3 cases and a mixed appearance in 2 cases.

2.brain CT

All patients had undergone a cerebral CT scan.

It enabled :

- Specify the number of lesions.
- Reveal a single lesion in all patients.
- Localize lesions.
- Specify size and determine density.

All the bones of the cranial vault were affected, with a clear predilection for the frontal and parietal bones.

The table below details the locations of the vault tumors in our series.

Table IIIDistribution of patients by cranial location

Topography	Number of cases	Percentage
Frontal bone	8	40%
Occipital bone	4	20%
Temporal bone	1	5%
Parietal bone	7	35%
Total	20	100%

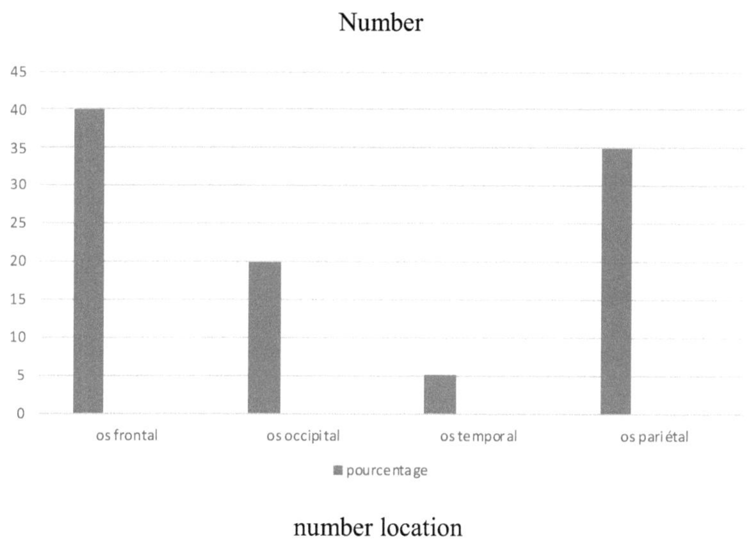

Figure 4Distribution of patients by cranial location

We noted a predominance of frontal localization with 8 cases (40%), followed by parietal localization with 7 cases (35%).

Temporal localization was found in only one case, i.e. 5% of cases in our series.

- Lesion size of :

    Size < 3 cm in 3 cases.

    Size between 3 and 5 cm in 14 cases.

    Size > 5 cm in 3 cases.

- Density :

The lesion was hyperdense in 7 cases, hypodense in 10 and mixed in 3.

3. Brain MRI

Eleven patients had undergone brain MRI, in addition to brain CT.

Brain MRI was used to study the tissue component, intracranial extension and sinus infiltration.

It showed 9 cases of tissue lesions and 2 cases of cystic lesions.

4. Bone scan

Four patients underwent bone scintigraphy as part of the extension work-up. It showed a single lesion in the vault in 3 cases, and foci of hyperfixation on the skeleton in 1 case.

5.cerebral angiography

Angiography was not performed in our patients.

Table IVDistribution of radiological examinations

Type of examination performed	Number of cases
Standard X-ray	7
CT SCAN	20
MRI	11
Angiography	0
Scintigraphy	4

6.Biology

All our patients underwent a biological work-up including a CBC, blood group, renal function, haemostasis and blood ionogram as part of their preoperative work-up.

Thyroid tests including FT4 and TSH were performed on two patients.

Tumor markers (PSA for 2 patients, ACE CA125, CA15-5) were detected in 9 patients:

An increase in PSA above 20 was noted in one patient.

A disturbance of the thyroid balance was observed in one patient.

The rest of the workup was normal.

Liver function tests (ASAT, ALAT) were carried out in both patients with histiocytosis X, and returned normal.

D. Treatment

Surgical excision was complete in 16 patients, and partial in 3.

Reconstruction was performed in 18 of our patients.

The dura mater was respected in all our patients except in two cases: One patient had infiltration of the superior sagittal sinus, which was ligated in its anterior third.

E.Histological examination

Histological examination was performed on all patients. This confirmed our suspicion with certainty.

The results were dominated by metastases in 7 cases, i.e. 35% of cases in our series: 2 cases from thyroid carcinoma, 2 cases from breast cancer, 1 case from prostate cancer, 1 case from bronchial cancer, 1 case from a local extension of a lacrimal gland tumor.

The majority of our patients were being followed for their primary cancer.

Only 2 cases were followed up in our department for vault swelling, and investigations and anatomopathological examination revealed the primary site.

Other histological types are :

- Four cases of osteoma
- Two cases of bone hemangiomas
- Two cases of histiocytosis X
- A case of neurofibroma
- A case of epidermoid cyst
- A case of intraosseous meningioma
- Two cases of primary malignant tumors:
  - ✓ A case of osteosarcoma
  - ✓ A case of chondrosarcoma

Table V Lesion distribution by pathological examination

	Nature of lesion	Histological nature	Number	Percentage
Primary tumors	Benign tumors	Osteoma	4	35%
		Hemangioma	2	
		Epidermoid cyst	1	
	Malignant tumors	Chondrosarcoma	1	10%
		Osteosarcoma	1	
	Pseudotumors and tumors of various origins	Histiocytosis x	2	20%
		Meningioma	1	
		Neurofibroma	1	
Secondary tumors	Metastases	Bronchial squamous cell carcinoma	1	35%
		Prostatic carcinoma	1	
		Thyroid cancer	2	
		Breast cancer	2	
	Local	Adenocarcinoma of the lacrimal gland	1	

F. Further treatment

Nine patients received additional treatment

One patient with osteosarcoma had received postoperative chemotherapy.

Patients with metastatic lesions were referred to a carcinology department.

G. Evolution

The short-term evolution was favorable for the majority of our patients.

The long-term evolution was favorable for 11 patients with benign lesions after a mean follow-up of 18 months.

On the other hand, those with malignant lesions had a fairly poor prognosis.

Three patients had experienced local recurrence.

Three patients died after a mean follow-up of 21 months.

II.Results by tumor type

A. Primary tumors

1.benign tumors

1.1. Osteomas

In our series we collected4 cases of osteomas in 2 men and 2 women, with an average age of 29 years.

- Clinical :

The mode of discovery common to all our patients was a swelling of the skull. Associated headache was found in 2 cases.

The time between the swelling and consultation was relatively long, with an average of 8 years and extremes ranging from 2 to 10 years.

Swelling sizes ranged from 2 to 4cm.

The lesions were located in :

-The frontal bone in 2 cases;

-Parietal bone in 2 cases.

One patient presented a recurrence after 9 months of surgical excision.

The notion of head trauma was found in 3 patients, i.e. 75% of cases.

- Imaging :

Skull X-rays in 2 patients showed well-limited, rounded opacities with a calcium tone.

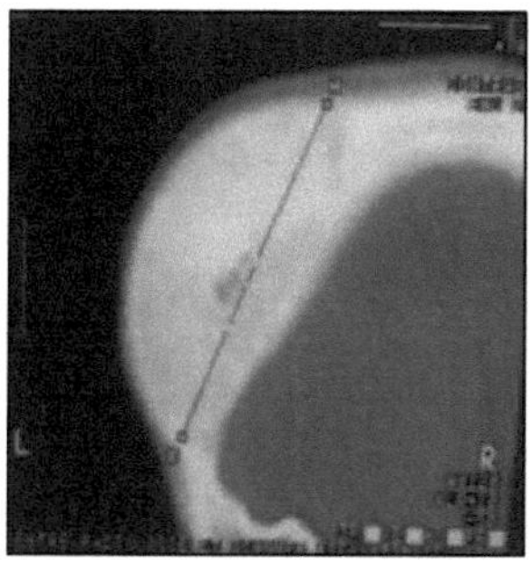

Figure 5(Obs 12) osteoma: brain CT: left frontal osteocondensation

Cerebral CT scans in our 4 patients confirmed the presence of a dense, homogeneous lesion and clarified its boundaries.

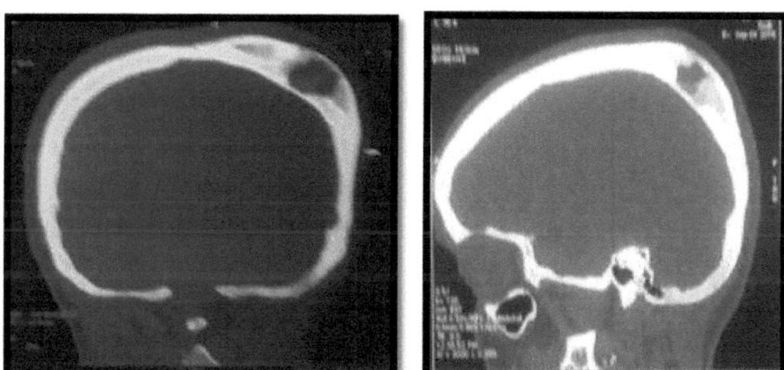

Figure 6 (obs12)

Cerebral CT in coronal(a) and sagittal(b) reconstruction: intradipoidal bone lesion of the left parietal convexity of mixed osteo-condensing and lytic appearance, 5*2 cm.

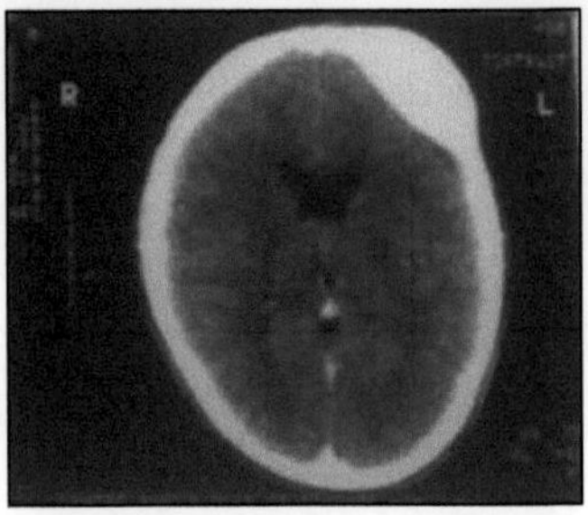

Figure 7Cerebral CT axial section: voluminous left frontal condensing lesion with respect for the medial cortex.

- Processing :

All our patients had undergone complete surgical excision of the lesion and concomitant cranioplasty.

One patient presented a recurrence of the lesion at the same surgical site with a delay of 9 months, necessitating repeat surgery which was complicated intraoperatively by an accidental tear of the dura mater.

In the immediate postoperative period she presented with a generalized convulsive seizure.

She was admitted to the intensive care unit for 24-hour monitoring.

- Pathological examination :

In all four patients, the surgical specimen was for pathological examination. This revealed trabeculae of haversian compact bone and multiple invasculo-adipal spaces with clear lesion boundaries.

- Evolution :

With a 3-year follow-up, all patients had a favorable outcome.

1.2. Intraosseous meningiomas

The patient was 52 years old, with no previous pathological history, and had consulted us for a right parietal swelling, more or less soft, painless, appearing 64 months previously and evolving slowly, associated with headaches.

- Imaging :

X-rays of the skull *showed* a homogeneous segmental osteocondensing lesion.

Non-injection and post-injection *CT* showed localized thickening and homogeneous densification of the diploe's outer lamina, with the inner lamina irregular.

MRI confirmed the presence of a tissue process arising in the right parietal cranial vault, fairly well limited and with an intra-diploid origin.

- *Processing* :

Treatment consisted of wide surgical resection under general anaesthetic, with immediate cranioplasty. The post-operative course was straightforward

- Anatomopathological examination :

Anatomopathological examination concluded that the tumor was an intraosseous meningioma made up of epithelial-like cells grouped into islands separated from each other by a thin conjunctivo-vascular tissue, reminiscent of the stroma of neuroendocrine tumors. Tumor cells had sparse cytoplasm and round nuclei with fine chromatin that resembled one another.

On immunohistochemical examination, the tumor cells focally expressed the epithelial markers Cytokeratin and EMA.

- Evolution :

Progression was favourable after a 2-year follow-up.

1.3. Hemangiomas

We collected 2 cases of hemangiomas in 1 man and 1 woman, with an average age of 30 years.

- Clinical :

This lesion was discovered following the onset of cranial swelling in 1 patient and headaches in 1 patient.

The time to consultation was 6 months and 3 years, and the swelling was parietal in one case and frontal in the other, measuring approximately 2 cm in both patients.

- Imaging :

Skull radiography was performed in 1 patient, showing an opacity at the expense of the parietal bone.

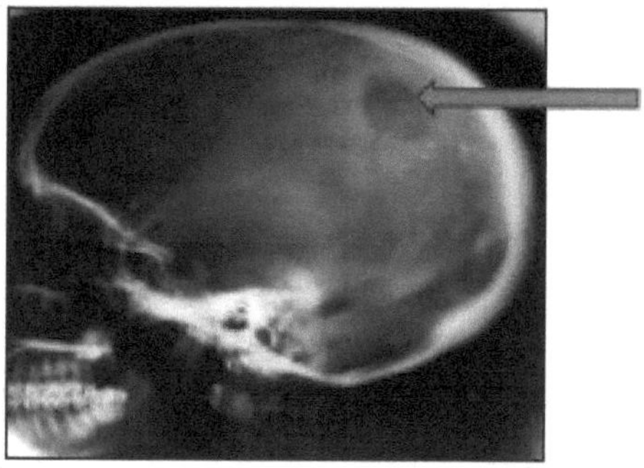

Figure 8(Obs. 10): Bone hemangioma. Skull X-ray: osteolytic lesion of the left parietal bone (arrow).

CT scans were performed in our 2 patients, and led to the diagnosis of hemangioma.

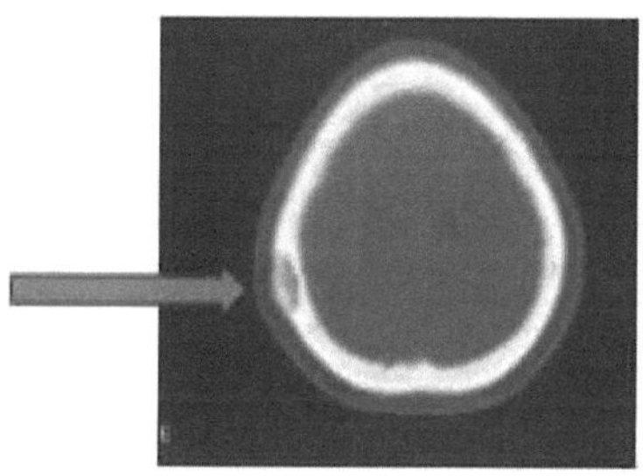

Figure 9(Obs. 10): Bone hemangioma: cerebral CT in axial section, image of right parietal osteolysis on the bone window.

- Processing :

Complete removal of the lesion was achieved in the 2patients with immediate cranioplasty.

Postoperative management was straightforward in these 2 patients.

- *Pathological examination* :

Pathological examination was carried out in both patients. This confirmed the diagnosis, showing a benign vascular tumor formed by the proliferation of capillary-type vascular structures, lined by a regular endothelium. These structures are separated by sparsely cellular fibrous tissue. The tumor was surrounded on the surface by a thick fibrous capsule that extended into bundles of striated muscle cells.

- Evolution :

After a mean follow-up of 9 months, all patients had a favourable outcome with no complications or recurrences.

1.4. Neurofibroma

- Clinic

This was a 51-year-old patient who had consulted for moderate headaches for 3 years without signs of intracranial hypertension.

Examination revealed a soft, painful, non-inflammatory left latero-occipital swelling measuring 6 cm long.

- Imaging

Standard radiography was not performed.

Cerebral CT showed a tumoral process involving the left occipital bone, with extracranial extension and bone destruction. The mass was tissue-dense, well bounded by a hyperdense wall with punctiform calcifications. The mass was intra-diploid, heterogeneous, with central necrosis and intense peripheral contrast (FIGURE 10).

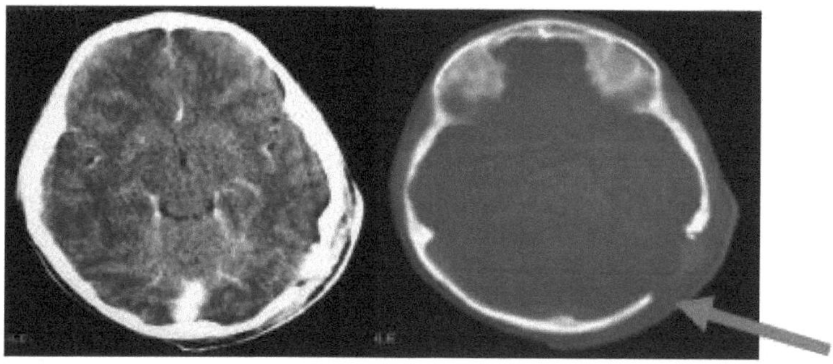

Figure 10(Obs. 1): Neurofibroma. Cerebral CT: Tumoral process in the left occipital bone, with extracranial extension and bone destruction in bone window sections.

Cerebral MRI showed a heterogeneous lesion process with hyposignal on SpT1, SpT2 and Flair, associating a necrotic central liquid zone with a fleshy peripheral zone strongly enhanced by Gadolinium.

- Processing :

The patient had undergone monobloc surgical excision of a partially cystic fleshy process; with bone reconstruction at the same operative time.

- Pathological examination :

Histopathological examination concluded that the tumor was proliferating with spindle-shaped cells arranged in bundles on a fibro-hyaline background. Immunohistochemistry revealed tumour cell labelling with PS100 and vimentin. All suggestive of a neurofibroma.

- Evolution :

Progression is good with a 5-year follow-up.

1.5 Epidermoid cysts

The patient was 42 years old, with no notable pathological history.

- Clinical :

She was admitted for a frontal swelling that had appeared 5 years ago, with a progressive increase in the size of the lesion and recent localized headaches without vomiting or seizures. The swelling was painless, 3 cm long, soft, non-pulsatile, fixed in relation to the deep planes, mobile in relation to the superficial planes and without inflammatory signs. The rest of the examination was unremarkable.

- Imaging :

Standard radiography: revealed a bony lacuna involving the roughly rounded, well-limited frontal arch, encircled by a fine line of condensation.

Computed tomography (CT) confirmed this mass as a homogeneous liquid hypodensity (between 12 and 25 Hounsfield Units) with a few calcifications inside. Intradiploid in location, this process was responsible for destruction of the external and internal tables without endocranial extension, did not take up contrast medium and the cerebral parenchyma opposite showed no pathological character (Fig. 11).

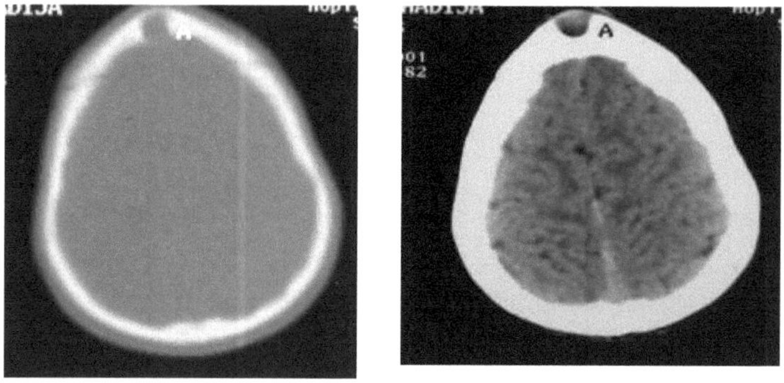

Figure 11(Obs.4): Epidermoid cyst: cerebral CT: well-circumscribed hypodense intra-diploid lesion of both bony tables, the location and appearance suggest an epidermoid or dermoid cyst.

On magnetic resonance imaging (MRI), the process was well limited, iso-hyposignal on T1-weighted sequences and hypersignal on T2-weighted sequences, compressing the brain parenchyma without any signs of brain invasion, as evidenced by a fine T2-hyposignal separation line. On coronal section, the scalp was not infiltrated. In the FLAIR sequence, the contents of the process were heterogeneous in signal, different from that of the cerebrospinal fluid (CSF). No gadolinium injection was performed.

- Processing :

The surgical procedure involved an arciform, inferiorly hinged skin incision centred on the process, followed by scalp detachment. This revealed a thin, cleavable capsule under tension, which had been weakened during dissection, releasing a more or less thick liquid content associated with pseudomembranous formations and pearly whitish lamellae: an appearance highly suggestive of an epidermoid cyst. The tumor capsule was completely removed, and a cranioplasty of the defect was performed using acrylic cement. Post-operative management was straightforward.

- Anatomopathological examination :

Histological study confirmed the epidermoid nature of the cyst, with no degenerative character.

- Evolution :

Clinical evolution is good after 3 years.

1.6. Histiocytosis X

Two cases of histiocytosis X with an average age of 35 years were reported in two patients with no notable pathological history.

- Clinical :

A patient presented with a parietal swelling 4 cm in diameter, progressively increasing in size and evolving for 2 months, associated with headaches.

The second patient had consulted for atypical headaches.

- Imaging :

In the first patient, *the brain scan* showed a voluminous left parietal condensing lesion with bone lysis of the vault opposite, and in the second patient, the CT scan showed a heterogeneous lytic lesion.

Cerebral MRI revealed a tissue lesion, with bone lysis of the vault opposite in both patients.

- Processing :

The procedure involved monobloc surgical excision by craniectomy of a grayish, patchy necrotic, pithy and slightly hemorrhagic tumor.

A cranioplasty was performed. The post-operative course was straightforward.

- Anatomopathological examination :

Anatomopathological examination revealed a mass formed by the proliferation of langerhansian histiocytic cells, characterized by more or less abundant eosinophilic cytoplasm and, above all, by crumpled or incised nuclei.

These cells were focally associated with multinucleated giant cells and, above all, with eosinophilic polymorphs. The tumor showed extensive foci of necrosis.

The bone fragments examined involved cortical bone and were infiltrated by Langerhansian cells. Immunohistochemical study showed intense nuclear and cytoplasmic positivity of most cells with anti-protein

S100(PS100), and cytoplasmic positivity with anti CD1a.

Anti CD68a was positive for some of these cells, especially multinucleated cells.

These results supported the diagnosis of Langerhansian histiocytosis.

- Evolution :

An extension work-up, including a thoraco-abdomino-pelvic CT scan and a biological work-up, had proved normal, hence the decision not to treat.

Progression was favourable after a 1-year follow-up.

2. Malignant bone tumors

2.1. Osteosarcoma

This was a 23-year-old patient with no notable pathological history.

➤ Clinical :

The patient had presented for 5 months with a left temporo-parieto-occipital tumefaction, soft fixed, painful polylobed without inflammatory signs opposite with a size of 3cm/2.

➤ Imaging:

Skull X-ray: not performed

Cerebral CT: revealed a tumoral process of the vault, with heterogeneous calcifications associated with endocranial extension. (Fig. 12).

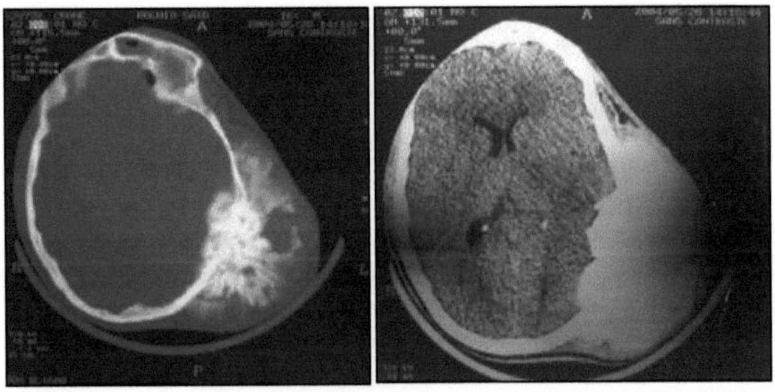

Figure 12(Obs.5): Cerebral CT osteosarcoma: huge tumoral process of the cranial vault with heterogeneous calcifications (a) associated with endocranial extension (b).

➢ Processing :

Treatment consisted of subtotal excision of the lesion.

➢ Anatomopathological examination :

The various tumor fragments were cribriform in appearance, including bone-adherent tissue corresponding to a highly cellular malignant tumor. Tumor cells had sparse cytoplasm, sometimes eosinophilic, sometimes clear, and showed moderate nuclear atypia and fairly numerous mitoses (8 mitoses/10fields at high magnification).

These cells surrounded thin, small osteoid trabeculae, some of which were surrounded by osteoid substance. Some osteoid trabeculae were calcified. (Fig. 13).

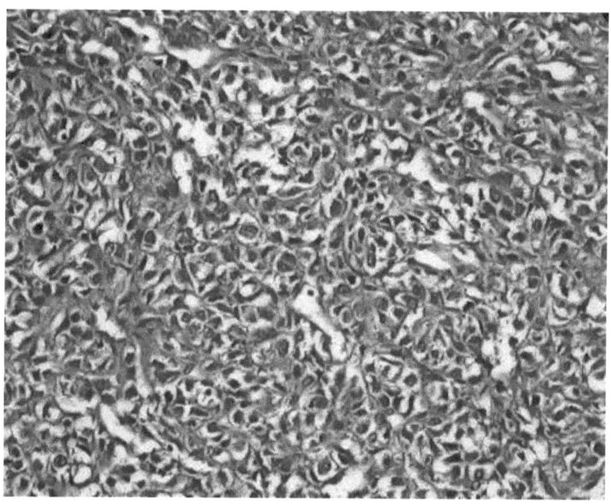

Figure 13(Obs. 5): Osteosarcoma. Malignant tumour proliferation rich in atypia with small osteoid trabeculae (hematoxilin and eosin, high magnification).

➤ Further treatment and development :

A chest CT scan performed as part of the extension work-up was normal. The decision was then taken to undertake 2 courses of chemotherapy followed by adjuvant radiotherapy.

Patient died after 5 months with local recurrence.

2.2 Chondrosarcoma

➤ Clinic

A 20-year-old young man with no previous history consulted initially for a left retro-auricular swelling. Neurological examination was unremarkable.

➤ Imaging:

The CT scan showed an extracranial centimetric cystic lesion developing on the outer table of the temporo-occipital synchondrosis. (Fig.14).

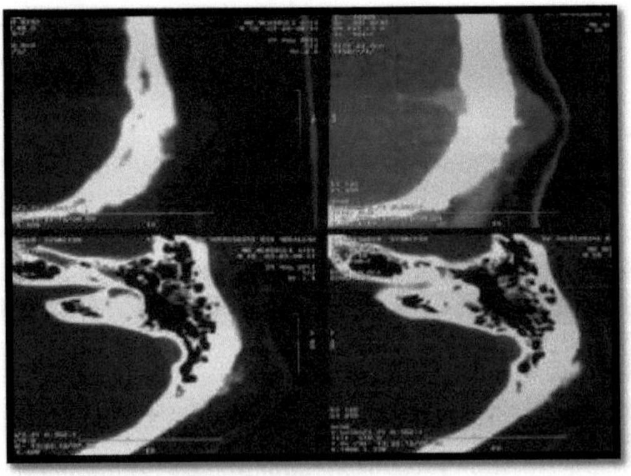

Figure 14 (obs 11):a) chondrosarcoma Brain CT: axial section through bone and parenchymal window

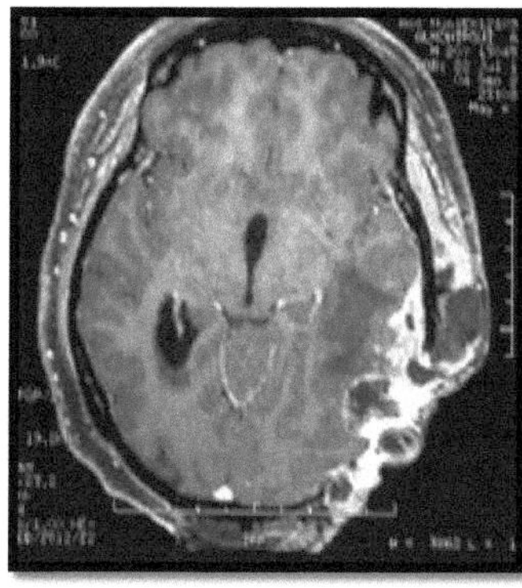

b) T2-sequence brain MRI after 2 years of evolution

- Processing :

A cytopunction was performed first, followed by incomplete tumor resection.

- Anatomopathological study :

Concluded that it was a grade I chondrosarcoma.

- Adjuvant treatment and evolution :

The lesion recurred at 03 months post-operatively, necessitating further surgery.

Radiotherapy at a dose of 50 Gy was attempted. The patient recurred on 2 further occasions, requiring the same number of surgical procedures, including a partial craniectomy. After 4 months from the last recurrence, he was seen again for headaches and dizziness, with a mixed cerebellar syndrome on examination.

By this time, the tumor had invaded the left cerebellar and parietal brain parenchyma and had become inoperable.

The patient died 02 months later.

B. Secondary tumors: Cranial metastases

Our series included 7 cases of cranial vault metastases with an average age of 65 years.

- *Clinical* :

The mode of discovery was a swelling in 5 patients associated with headaches.

Discovery was fortuitous in two cases.

Neurological examination was unremarkable.

- Imaging :

X-rays of the skulls of two patients showed bone lysis.

Cerebral CT scans revealed osteolytic lesions in all 7 cases.

In one patient, brain *MRI* revealed infiltration of the superior sagittal sinus.

The scintigraphy performed on4 patients showed :

For a patient diagnosed with breast carcinoma: multiple foci of hyperfixation in the occipito parietal cranial vault, left greater trochanter and left ischium.

On the basis of radiological and pathological examinations, the diagnosis was breast carcinoma with bone metastases.

In the other three patients, scintigraphy was normal except for lesions in the arch.

- Processing :

In view of the advanced stage of the disease, 2 patients abstained from treatment, while 5 underwent surgical excision.

- Evolution :

Two patients died with an average delay of 7 months.

The other patients were referred to their oncologists for follow-up.

Table VI Summary table of patients with metastatic lesions

Gender Age(years)	History	Discovery mode	Clinical examination	Paraclinical examination	Treatment	Anapath	Post-operative care	Evolution
F/ 62	Dyslipidemia Mammary carcinoma	Parieto-occipital swelling	Painful, non-inflammatory parieto-	X-ray: lytic lesion CT: osteolytic lesion Scintigraphy: multiple	Abstention	-	-	Deceased

			occipitalen on tumefaction, 5/4 cm in size	secondary locations				
F/ 54	Mammary carcinoma	A chance discovery	Headaches	CT: 2 cm frontal osteolytic lesion Scintigraphy: single lesion of the arch	Total removal + cranioplasty	Mammary carcinoma	Simple	Good progress
H/ 67	Cataract surgery Total thyroidectomy+iodotherapy	Left frontal swelling	Left frontal swelling, 5 cm in diameter, soft, firm, painless, attached to deep planes	Skull X-ray: lacunar image of the frontal bone With peripheral osteocondensation CT: external endocranial bone lesion	Total excision iodotherapy	Metastasis of vesicular thyroid carcinoma	Simple	Favorable
H / 59	RAS	Forehead swelling	Fixed, painless 4	MRI: underlying osteolysis tissue mass	Total excision	Vesicular carcinoma	Simple	Favorable

			cm frontal swelling, 3 cm hard cervical mass	and infiltration of the upper sagittal sinus				
H/46	Treated pulmonary TBK	Incidental discovery during the workup of a cough and hemoptysis		TDM : Bone lysis of the arch involving the outer and inner table	Total excision	Bone metastasis of poorly differentiated squamous cell carcinoma	Surgical site superinfection	Lost from sight
H/68	Prostatic carcinoma	AEG Left frontal swelling	Irregular hard left fronto-parietal swelling with	MRI: extracranial swelling with osteolysis	Surgical biopsy	Metastasis of vesicular carcinoma	Simple	Passed away

			out inflammatory signs					
F/70	Operated adenocarcinoma of the lacrimal gland	Headaches	Forehead swelling	TDM :	Subtotal excision	Local metastasis	Simple	Stable

Illustration of some cases of patients with secondary lesions

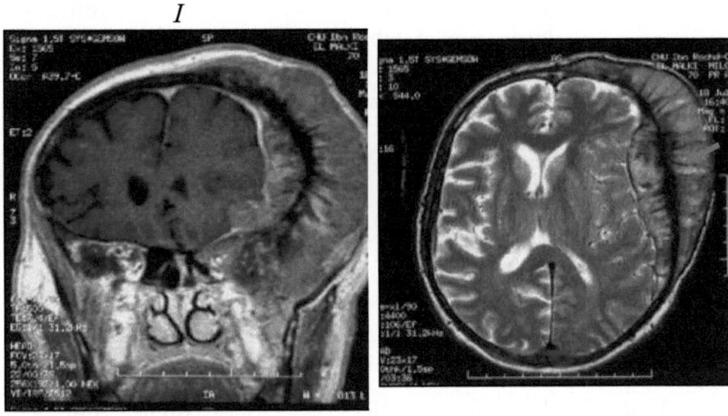

Figure 15(Obs. 2): Bone metastasis of prostatic carcinoma. Cerebral MRI in T1 coronal section showing an isointense signal lesion occupying the extradural space and soft tissues with bone destruction (a). In T2 axial section, the lesion retains the same signal (b).

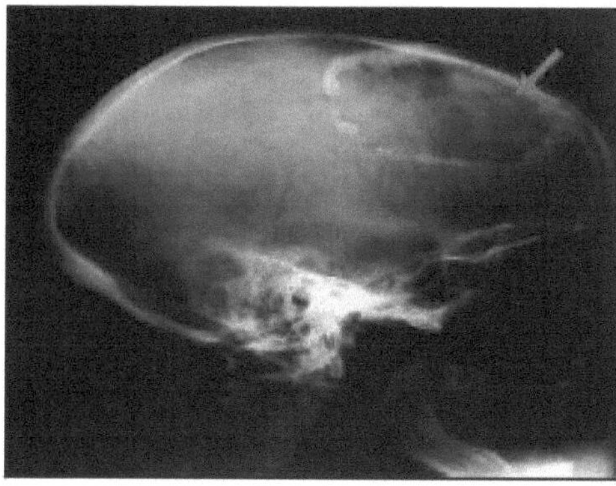

Figure 16(Obs.3): Bone metastases from thyroid carcinoma. Skull X-ray: Lacunar image over the left frontal bone with peripheral osteocondensation.

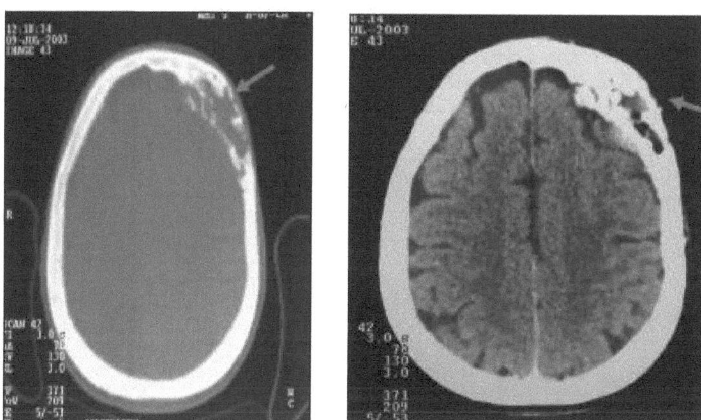

Figure 17(Obs. 4): Bone metastases of thyroid carcinoma: cerebral CT in axial sections in bone window (a) and parenchymal window (b): aggressive fronto-parietal bone lesion blowing and destroying the diploea and both external and internal tables, with discrete pericerebral endocranial extension without parenchymal invasion.

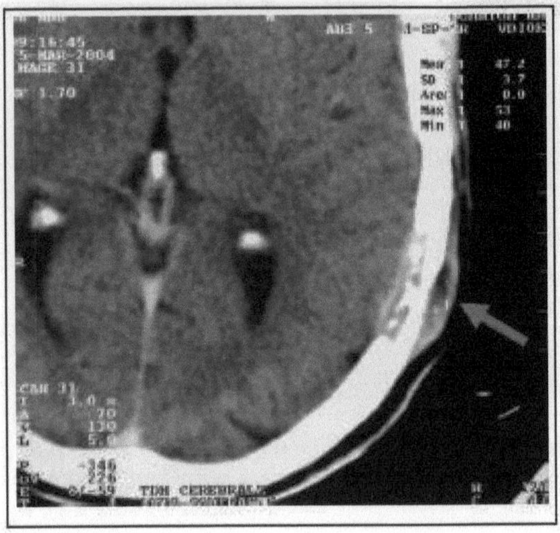

Figure 18(Obs. 4): Bone metastases from bronchial carcinoma. CEREBRAL CT: axial section in parenchymal window: left posterior parietal bone lysis of the vault involving a completely lysed inner table and a nibbled outer table.

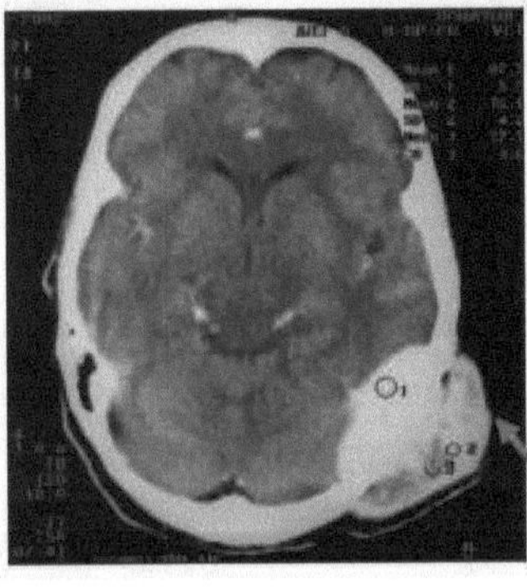

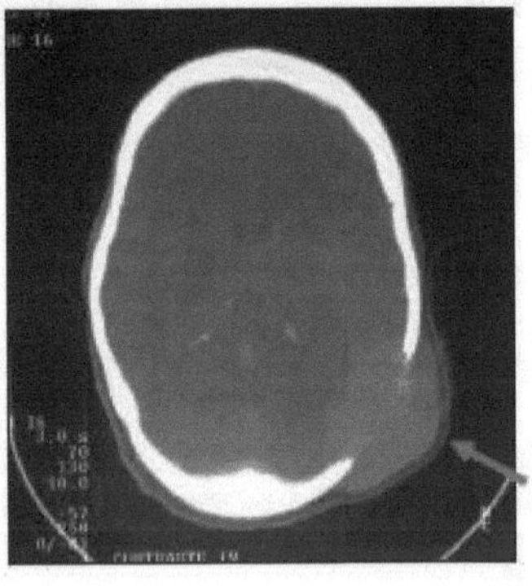

Figure 19(Obs.6): Bone metastases from thyroid carcinoma: CEREBRAL CT:Left occipital cranial tumour process, with intracranial extension, associated with massive contrast-enhancing bone lysis.

a)

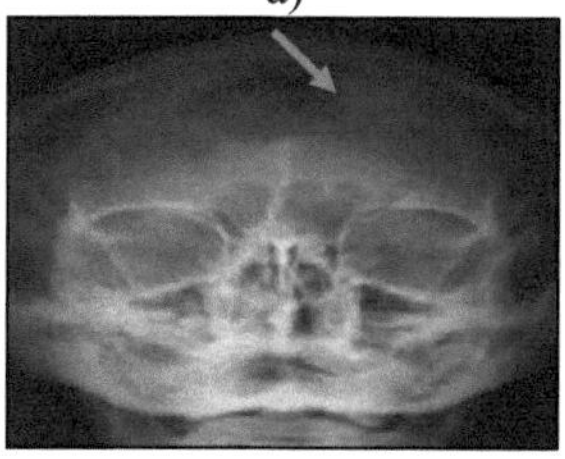

b)

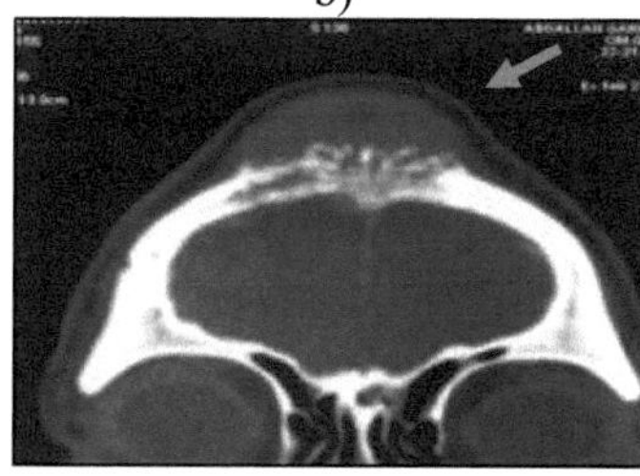

c)

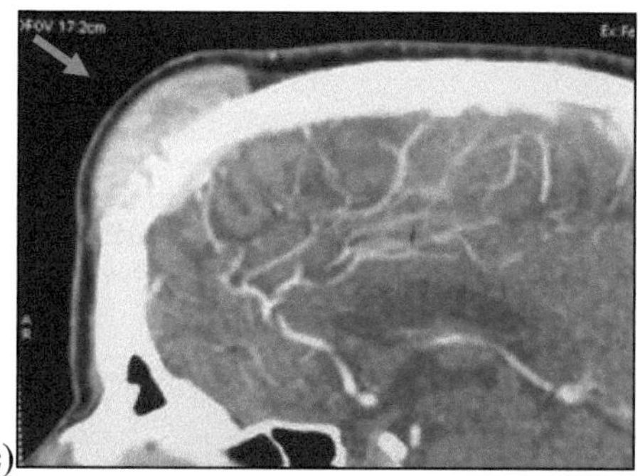

Figure 20. Obs :13. a) X-ray of the skull showing a frontal lytic lesion b) CT brain coronal section showing an osteolytic lesion with destruction of the medial cortex c) sagittal reconstruction section showing infiltration of the superior sagittal sinus

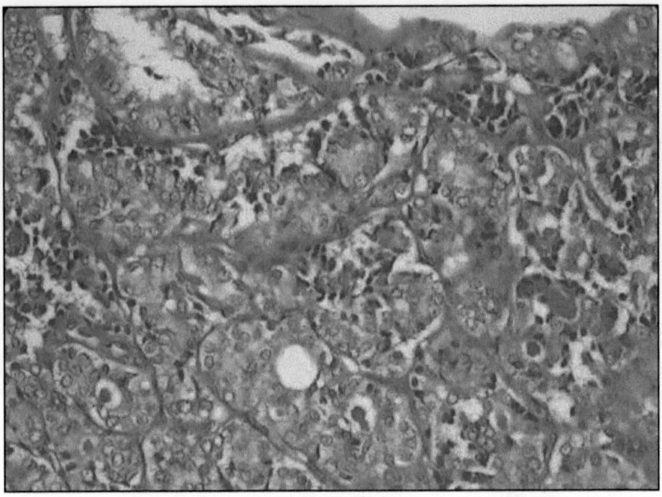

Figure 21(Obs. 3): Thyroid bone metastases. At higher magnification, the vesicles are lined by a tumoral coating, with lumina sometimes containing colloid material (hematoxylin and eosin at high magnification).

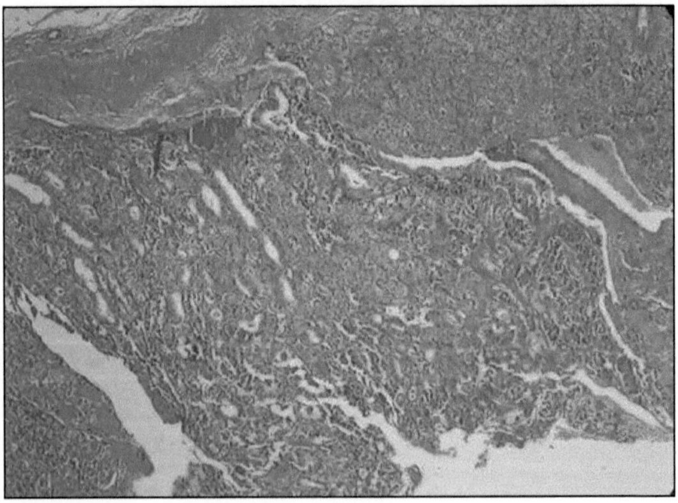

Figure 22(Obs. 3): Thyroid bone metastases. Side view, vesicular tumor (hemathein and eosin, low magnification).

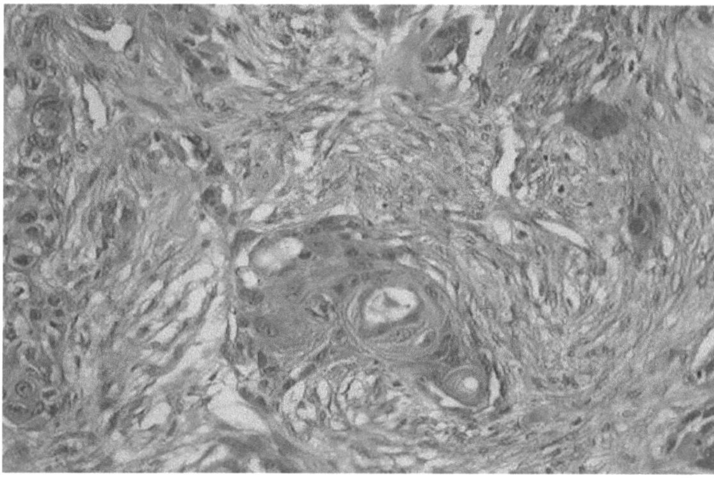

Figure 23(Obs. 4): Bone metastases from bronchial squamous cell carcinoma. Squamous tumour proliferation arranged in casings around a focus of dyskeratosis (hematoxylin and eosin, high magnification).

Observation 9: Surgical removal of a frontal lesion of the arch

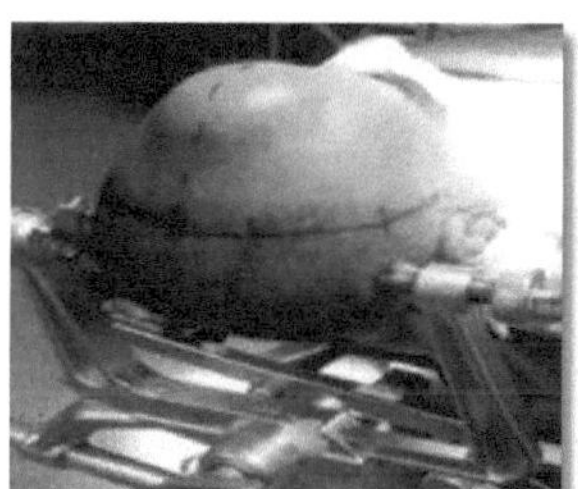

Figure 24 Patient positioning

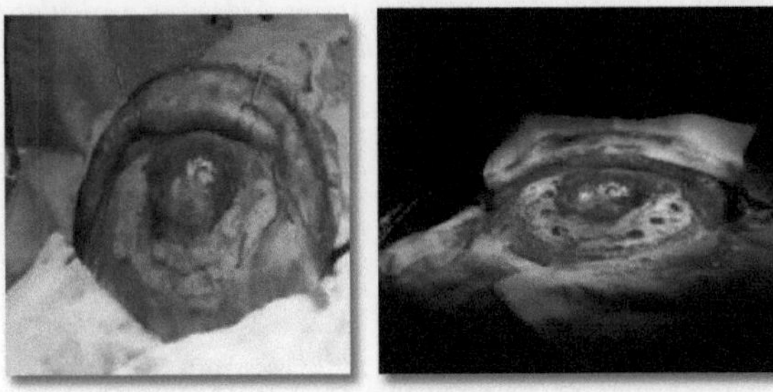

Figure 25 a) Dark red fleshy lesion adherent to the deep plane b) Bone flap made with drill holes

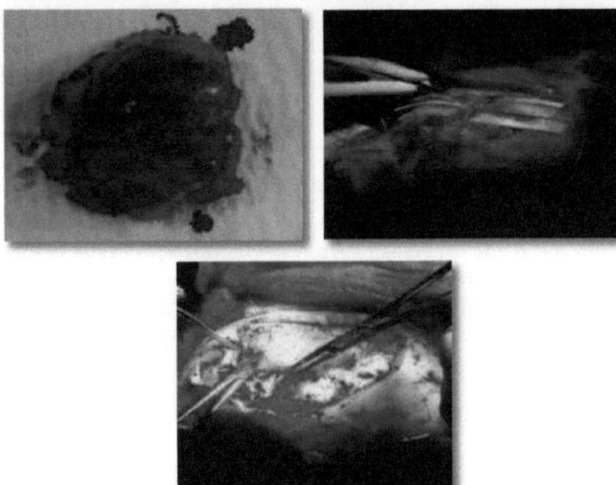

Figure 26 En bloc excision of the lesion and ligation of the SSS

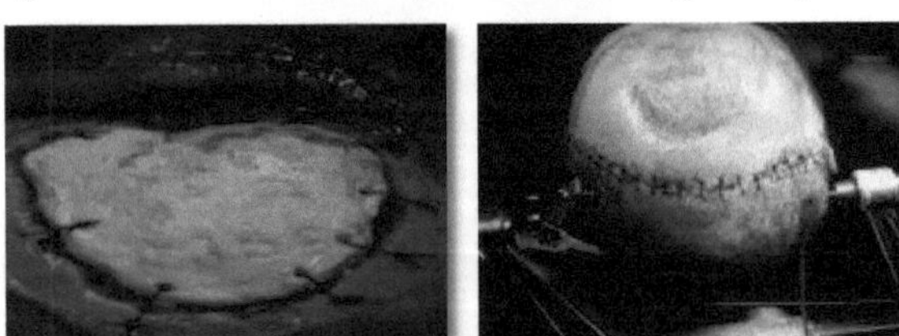

Figure 27:Cranioplasty and skin closure

DISCUSSION

I. Primary tumors

A. Benign tumors

1. Epidermoid cyst

It remains asymptomatic for a long time, due to its extremely slow progression. Neurological disorders are exceptional, although some frontal localizations may manifest as exophthalmos. The swelling is generally small and firm.[1,2,3].

In our series, a patient with an epidermoid cyst presented with isolated frontal localized swelling.

1.1 Epidemiology

- Frequency :

Formerly known as pearl tumors or cholesteatomas

First described by CRUVEILHIER in 1829, it accounts for less than 1% of all intracranial tumours.[1,2].

Its location in the vault of the skull accounts for 25% of all epidermoid cysts[4].

- Location:

In the cranial vault, it is mainly located in the frontal and parietal bones, particularly near the coronal suture, although all other locations are possible. [5,6].

- Age/sex-ratio :

It usually affects adults between the ages of 20 and 60, but can be observed at any age, with extremes ranging from 7 months to 87 years.[7].

1.2 Radiology

- Standard radiography:

Shows a single, rounded lacuna with sharp edges surrounded by marginal sclerosis localized near a suture. In more than 50% of cases, it is fronto-parietal, close to the coronal suture. When at a distance from a suture, it is often located on the occipital or temporal scales. Epidermoid cysts are more lateral than dermoid cysts. The size of the lacuna is variable, usually between 0.5 and 3 cm, but can sometimes be larger, up to 15 cm, giving a puffy image preferentially affecting the external table.

- CT :

The epidermoid cyst is liquid.

After injection, there is no contrast of the cyst contents.

- MRI:

Epidermoid cysts usually have a signal very close to that of cerebrospinal fluid in the different weightings, sometimes with linear enhyposignal trabeculae, sometimes concentric. The signal is not always strictly liquid and depends on its chemical composition. Peripheral contrast is common in epidermoid cysts, and absent in dermoid cysts.[8,9].

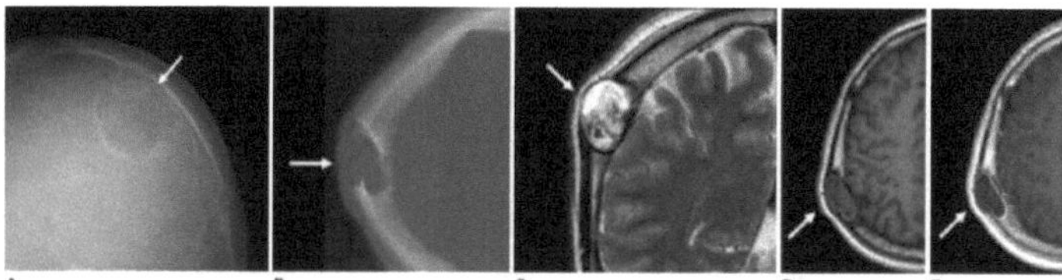

Figure 28 Epidermoid cyst on radiograph and axial section CT: circumscribed osteolytic lacuna surrounded by marginal sclerosis (A-B) on MRI coronal section T2

Heterogeneous appearance(C) hypointense T1 uninjected appearance(D) slight T1 contrast (E)[10]

1.3 Histology

Formerly called "pearl tumor" or cholesteatoma, the epidermoid cyst is a benign tumor of embryonic origin, resulting from a disorder of organogenesis. The epidermoid cyst can be primitive by inclusion of ectodermal embryonic debris during the development of bone outlines, or secondary to a traumatic inclusion of the epidermis.[3,7,11,12,13].

- Macroscopy :

The tumor is nippled with a pearly appearance, giving rise to CRUVEILHIER's "pearl tumor"; there is a peri-cystic reaction giving rise to an inflammatory granuloma.

- Microscopy :

It is a tumor made of squamous, squamous, well-differentiated, stratified, keratinized epithelium, with internal exfoliation, with desiccated, keratinized cell clusters, arranged in concentric strata in three layers:

- Conjunctive.

- Stratified epithelial.

- Cellular squamous.

Cholesterin is frequently present in the center, and keratohyalin granules are seen.

➤ Immunohistochemistry:

Epidermoid cyst surface epithelium is immunoreactive to cytokeratin and epithelial membrane antigen.

Malignant degeneration into squamous cell carcinoma is very rare. [14]Yanai et al. in [13,15,16]reported 13, including 3 in the skull vault. According to this author, this degeneration is due to multiple interventions, since in these 3 cases the malignant degeneration developed on recurrences.

1.4. Processing

In the case of epidermoid cysts, surgery removes the cyst and prevents recurrence. The tumour capsule, which forms the germinative part of the cyst, must be removed. This radical cure is usually only possible in the variety that does not adhere to the dura mater, the problem being completely different in the case of intracranial extension.[11,12,17]. It should be noted that for some authors, any discovery of an epidermoid cyst should result in surgical excision in order to prevent any subsequent complications [18].

2. Osteoma

Osteomas are most often asymptomatic and are discovered by chance. When present, the swelling is localized, with a consistency identical to that of the surrounding bone. Giant sinus osteomas destroy the sinus walls and are responsible for complications such as exophthalmos, optic atrophy, pneumatocele and meningitis. Multiple localizations are rare, and may form part of Gardner syndrome: an autosomal dominant hereditary condition associating cranial osteomas with rectocolic polyposis, gastric adenoma, congenital hypertrophy of the pigmented retinal epithelium and a skin cyst.[19,20,21].

2.1. Epidemiology

- Frequency :

According to VIRCHOW, it accounts for 20% of primary cranial vault tumors.

According to DANDY, they are by far the most common indigenous tumors of the skull. In our series, osteomas were found in 4 observations, representing 30% of the primary tumours in our series and 20% of all lesions.[19,10].

Osteomas grow very slowly, and usually take a long time to develop. In our series, the average time to diagnosis was 6 years.

Most osteomas remain asymptomatic and are discovered on radiological examination. However, they may be revealed by swelling, or headaches relieved by acetylsalicylic acid [9, 10]. Epistaxis and ophthalmological complications (ptosis, diplopia, etc.) have also been reported [9].

In our series, the common presenting sign was swelling, associated with headache in 3 cases.

Osteomas are generally small tumors, not exceeding 3 cm in long axis (11), but Kenneth et al reported a giant osteoma measuring 17.5 x 13.2 x 5 cm (11).

In our series, osteomas ranged in size from 2 to 4 cm.

- Location:

Osteomas occur almost exclusively in the craniofacial region, rarely in the long bones.

Osteomas are mainly located in the frontal and parietal regions, and more rarely in the temporal and occipital regions. In a study including 18 patients, William et al. reported parietal bone involvement as the most predominant [12].

In our series, the parietal bone was involved in 4 cases (44.4%), followed by the frontal bone in 3 cases.

On the cranial vault, it most often develops from the external table (exostosis); osteomas that develop from the internal table (enostosis) are exceptionally symptomatic.[19,10,22].

- Age/sex-ratio :

Osteomas can be observed at any age, but according to Chagnon et al they are mostly discovered during the 4ème - 5ème decades.[23],[24]. Most authors report a male preponderance, with a sex ratio ranging from 1.5 to 3.1 [4].

2.2. Radiology

Depending on the location in relation to the different layers of the skull vault and the direction of extension, three forms can be distinguished:

-exostosis

-intradiploid osteoma

- enostosis

2.2.1. Exostosis

This is the most common, and can be developed solely at the expense of the outer table.

- Standard radiography:

It is sufficient for diagnosis and shows a homogeneous hyperostosis of high density, which may be either extensive with a wide implantation base of 3 to 4 cm and thin thickness, or pedicled with short implantation[25].

- CT :

It shows whether or not the diploe is involved, with the internal table remaining normal or only slightly condensed.

The radiological appearance may be less typical when the osteoma is recent, in which case the hyperostosis is less homogeneous, containing a few spongy cavities. If the implant pedicle is still fibrous, the osteoma may appear falsely independent of the bone table[9].

2.2.2. Intradiploid osteoma

It is very rare, presenting on standard radiography as a rounded, homogeneous, well-limited hyperdensity, with no involvement of the bone tables.

2.2.3. Enostosis

It is rare, and above all difficult to differentiate from meningioma and any old calcified hematoma.

- Standard radiography:

The osteoma develops from the medial table and passes intracranially. The clear contour, homogeneous density and abrupt delineation with normal bone are criteria in favour of osteoma. There are no spicules or radiolucent bands between the vault and the mass.

In these three forms of vault osteoma, sutures are always respected and intra- and extra-cranial vascularization remains normal.

- CT :

it specifies the involvement of the bone tables, the homogeneous appearance of the mass and the repression of brain tissue[26,27].

- MRI:

The osteoma is homogeneous and hypointense in T1 and T2, with no enhancement after intravenous injection of gadolinium.

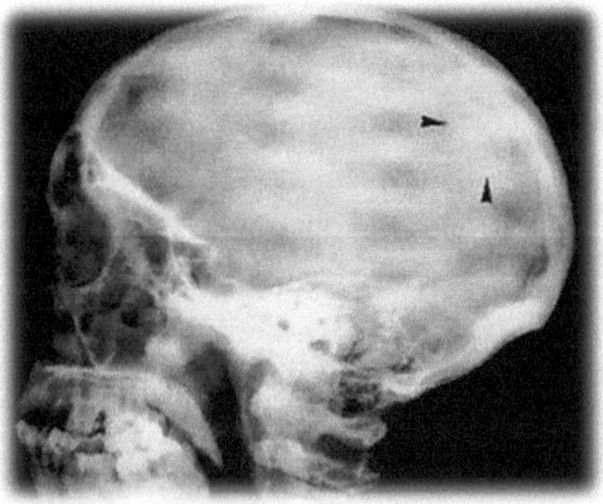

Figure 29Osteoma: profile skull X-ray showing a radiopaque mass Circumscribed left parietal bone[24].

2.3 Histology

The etiopathogenesis is still unknown, but three theories have been put forward:

□□□L embryological origin:

Proposed by Cohn Heim, this theory suggests that osteomas develop from residual embryonic remnants on the ethmoidal junction [4].

□□L of traumatic origin:

Championed by Gerber, this theory considers that trauma, especially during development, is involved in the genesis of osteomas [4].

□□L of infectious origin:

According to this theory, osteomas could have developed in areas of hypertrophy secondary to chronic bone infections [4].

Some authors have also suggested the role of abnormal bone development, neoplastic damage, lesions reactivated by trauma, muscle traction [6] or ossified fibrous dysplasia [7].

Skull vault osteomas are very dense, well limited and do not cross sutures [3].

In our series, 2 patients underwent skull radiography alone, 5 benefited from CT scans and 2 patients had both radiological examinations together.

In children, fibrous dysplasia (a less dense, less well-limited lesion most often found on the sphenoid and ethmoid bones) is the main differential diagnosis.

In adults, periosteal osteosarcoma should be considered, due to its severity (less clear contours, less dense and less homogeneous lesion) [9, 15, 16,17].

It is a benign tumour secondary to the elaboration of dense but normal bone from the periosteum and corresponds to the exaggeration of intra-membranous bone formation, it is made up of lamellar bone tissue, sometimes with areas of trabecular bone, there is no cartilaginous cap at its periphery [23].

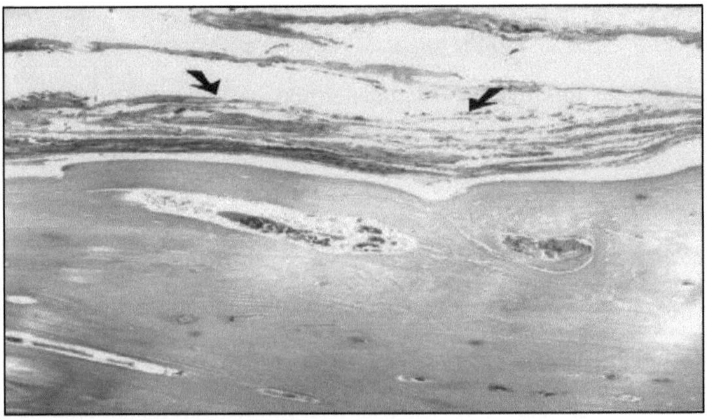

Figure 30Microscopic appearance of cranial osteoma: formed by mature lamellar bone surrounded by a fibrous membrane (dura mater). [28]

2.4. Treatment

The diagnosis of certainty will be confirmed by anatomopathological examination.

Treatment is often surgical. In the case of simple osteomas, treatment is based on en bloc resection or curettage of the tumour [11,18].

Abstention with annual radiological monitoring is the treatment of choice for osteomas that are strictly frontal, maxillary or ethmoidal in location, small, asymptomatic and without aesthetic prejudice [18], or in elderly patients [11].

The choice of surgical approach should take into account the location and extent of the osteoma, and possible complications [18].

Mugliston et al suggest that the same precautions proposed for malignant tumours in the same locations should be applied to the surgical treatment of osteomas (19, 20):

- Assessment of intracranial disease
- Brain protection
- Avoiding CSF leaks
- Correct hemostasis

Exeresis must be complete, with destruction of the tumor pedicle. It may be performed as a monobloc or by tumor fragmentation. The outer shell should be removed and the defect filled by cranioplasty [18].

According to some authors, recurrence after incomplete resection can reach10% of cases [21].

There are no cases of degeneration, but local post-operative complications have been reported by Chagnon et al (9).

In our series, all patients underwent complete surgical excision and cranioplasty.

3. Bone hemangioma

It is a rare lesion representing less than 1% of all bone tumors [32]. Bone hemangioma is a rare entity that is exceptionally associated with diffuse angiomatosis.

Identified by VIRKOW in 1864, bone hemangioma is a benign tumor of the hamartoma group.[29].

The bony mass is hard, palpable, solitary and slow-growing, with normal surrounding skin. In some cases, cholesteatoma-like symptoms may be observed in the petrous bone, with involvement of the VII and VIII cranial nerves.

Another unusual location is the orbit, where ptosis, strabismus and diplopia can occur. Hemorrhage is rare[30,31].

The most frequent mode of discovery is fortuitous during a radiological examination, more rarely clinical following the appearance of a hard, painless swelling covered by healthy skin adherent to the deep plane [34].

In our patients, 3 cases were revealed by a swelling, while only one case was discovered incidentally during a radiological examination.

In a review of the literature by Heckel et al (1975-2000), cranial hemangiomas mainly affected the frontal and temporal bones [33]. In our series, 2 cases were located in the parietal bone, one in the frontal bone and one in the parieto-occipital bone.

In general, there are no associated neurological signs, as the tumor grows very gradually without coming into contact with the brain parenchyma (intradiploid position) [34].

However, it may be accompanied by headaches and, depending on the location in the skull bones, exophthalmos in the case of orbital bone localization, or auditory signs in the case of localization in the external auditory canal [34].

3.1 Epidemiology

- Frequency :

Still known as diploid angioma, the first cranial hemangioma was reported in the literature by TOYBEE in 1845.

Its incidence is around 0.7 to 1% of all bone tumors, but this figure is underestimated, as evidenced by the frequency of chance discoveries[32,33].

The skull is affected second only to the spine, accounting for approximately 10% of all benign tumours of the cranial vault.[34,35]. Hemangiomas were found in two cases, i.e. 10% of cases in our series.

Cranial bony cavernous hemangiomas are even rarer, accounting for 0.2% of benign skull tumors [33, 34]. The first case was described by Toynbee in 1845 [33].

In a review of the literature from 1845 to 1981, Barnes described 123 cases of cranial bone hemangiomas [33]. In another review, Stephan et al presented 103 similar cases collected over 25 years (1975 to 2000) [33].

In our series, there were 4 cases of hemangiomas, representing 17.4% of all bone tumors and 26.7% of benign bone tumors.

- Location:

The vault of the skull, along with the vertebral bodies and ribs, represent the main locations.

In the skull, it can occur in any region, but mainly in the frontal and parietal bones, and less frequently in the occipital, temporal and petrous bones.[33]

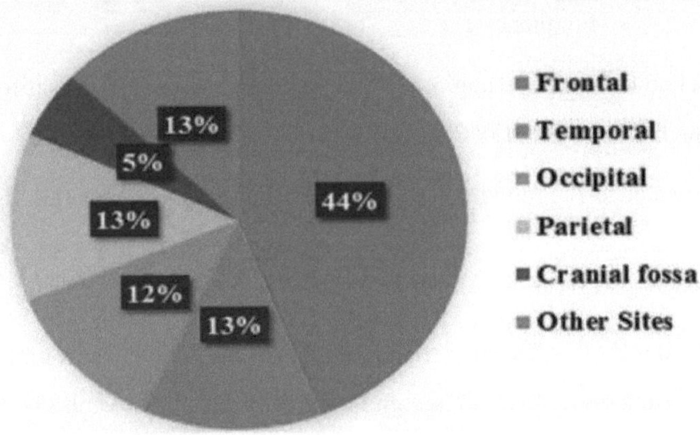

Figure 31:Location of intraosseous hemangiomas [36].

➢ Age/sex-ratio :

It was first discovered in adults during the 4-5ème decades, with a clear female predominance and a sex ratio of 1 male to 3 females.[33].

This tumor affects women in particular, and almost always young adults [34]. It occurs most frequently between the ages of 30 and 60, with extremes reported in the literature ranging from 1 month to 77 years [32].

In our series, there was no gender predominance, and the mean age of patients was 25.5 years, with extremes ranging from 4 months to 40 years.

Most of the cranial hemangiomas described have a single location [34], although there are cases of multiple locations [34].

In 2003, Erdogan et al described a case of multiple bony localization of cavernous angiomas involving the cranial vault and the 9ème rib, while Magnies et al described a case of multiple hemangiomas involving the cranial vault and liver [34].

3.2. Radiology

On imaging, standard radiographs most often show a sharp-edged, intradiploid, osteolytic lesion with a grid-like appearance, also known as a "honeycomb" [34].

Cerebral CT shows a lytic, limited intradiploiquebial lesion in the bone window, sometimes with erosion of the internal and/or external tables [34].

It allows us to study the location of the hemangioma and its relationship with adjacent structures [34].

Our four patients underwent CT scans which showed intradiploid lesions, with extension to the internal and external tables in two cases.

MRI usually shows an isointense lesion on T1-weighted imaging ethyper-intense onT2-weighted imaging, enhancing after gadolinium injection [34].

The classically heterogeneous appearance of the tumor is related to the presence of hemosiderin, methemoglobin, oxy and deoxyhemoglobin secondary to intra-tumoral hemorrhage [34].

The radiological appearance is not always specific, however, and there are numerous differential diagnoses, such as osteosarcoma, chondrosarcoma, metastases, multiple myeloma, meningioma, osteoma, Paget's disease, cholesteatoma, hyperparathyroidism, eosinophilic granuloma and epidermoid cyst [34].

- Standard radiography:

It shows a single, rounded lacuna, 1 to 7 cm in diameter, with clear boundaries, without peripheral condensation or with very fine marginal sclerosis. This diploid mass lifts and then erodes the outer table, while the inner table remains preserved for a long time. In general, there are no changes to the neighbouring diploid vessels.

Aspects suggestive of a bone hemangioma are :

-a heterogeneous beach, made up of spans forming a "breadcrumb" areolar image.

-Bone spicules within the lacuna and irregular, condensed margins give a "honeycomb" or "sunburst" appearance.

Plain radiography is the most widely used technique, especially for detecting the exact location of the lesion.

- CT :

It specifies the diploid location of the lesion, its effect on both the internal and external tables, and the appearance of the generally non-sclerotic margins. The lesion appears homogeneous with enhancement after PDC injection.[27,37,38].

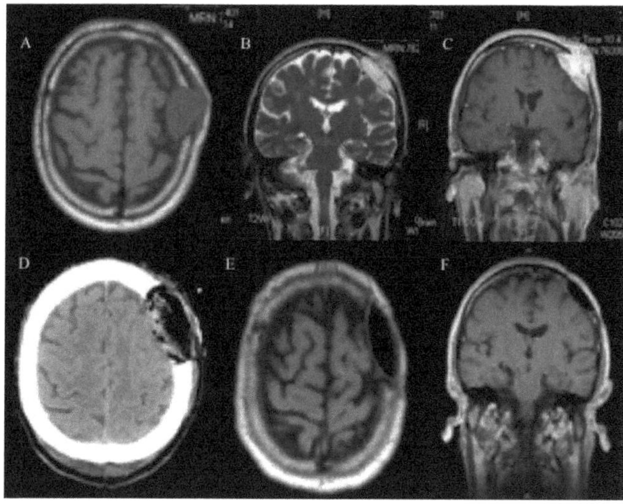

Figure 32 (A-C) Preoperative cerebral MRI reveals a large extra-axial lesion in the left frontal bone with intradural infiltration, predominantly T1-weighted axial (A), T2-weighted coronal hyperintense (B) and after gadolinium injection (C). (D) Postoperative cerebral CT shows disappearance of mass effect (E, F).

Gadolinium-weighted T1 axial and coronal MRI shows no recurrence.[39].

- MRI:

It shows an intraosseous tumor that is both isointense and hyperintense on the T1 signal, due to the existence of fine calcified trabeculae, and hyperintense on the T2 signal, which enhances intensely after gadolinium injection, due to the small size of the vascular channels and there is the absence of an identifiable outflow void that might suggest the vascular nature, of these lesions.

MRI is inferior to CT in the detection of bone destruction and in the study of cortical margins, whereas intradiploid and intracranial extension and invasion of vascular and neural structures are better detected by MRI. [38].

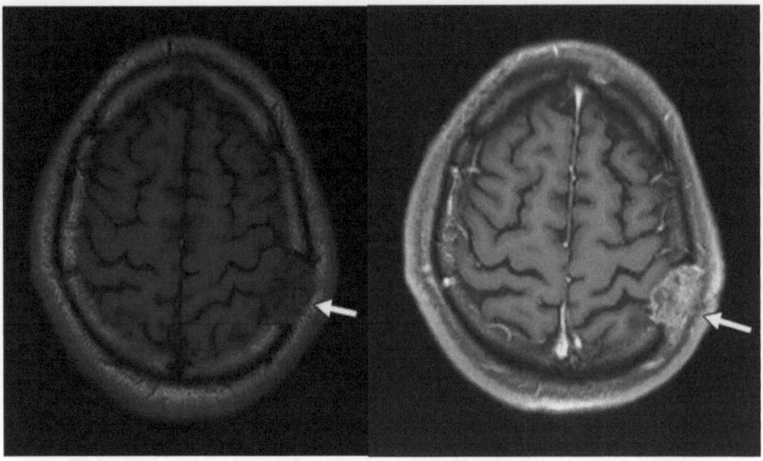

A B

Figure 33 A and B T1 axial cross-section brain MRI before and after gadolinium injection showing a single osteolytic lesion in the left parietal bone that is iso T1 intense(A) and contrast-enhancing after injection(B). [40].

- Angiography:

This is not a routine examination; it shows a hyper-vascular lesion, the drainage veins may be dilated but of normal size and contour. The angiographic results also help determine the possibility of preoperative embolization to reduce intraoperative blood loss in the case of hypervascularized hemangiomas. The hemangioma is fed by branches of the external carotid artery.

Bone scintigraphy: not very useful[35].

3.3 Histology

Intraosseous hemangioma is a benign primary lesion of the bone, characterized by the neoformation and agglomeration of abnormal blood vessels [32].

Hemangiomas can result from poor differentiation of the primordial vessels, giving an abnormal capillary bed.

- Macroscopy :

The tumor is fleshy (brown or red), consisting of cystic spaces, containing typical bone trabeculae, which explains the "honeycomb" radiological appearance; the tumor is vascularized with involvement of the internal or external table; extension of the tumor to the soft tissues can be seen[19,39,41,42].

- Microscopy :

Hemangiomas were classified:

Capillaries: these are enlarged masses of blood-filled sinusoidal channels that expose and displace normal tissue. The bone trabeculae seen in these tumors are the result of osteoclastic remodeling and osteoblastic reinforcement, in response to the conflict created by the tumor.

Venous: these contain a mixture of thick-walled venous channels, capillaries and arterioles, or bulky feeder vessels lined with endothelial cells.

-Cavernous: made up of large vessels and sinuses embedded in a connective matrix.

Cavernous histology is predominant in cranial hemangiomas.

In a review by PAILLAS et al, a few rare atypical forms were described (lacunar, pseudomeningiomatous, hyperostotic). [31,41,43].

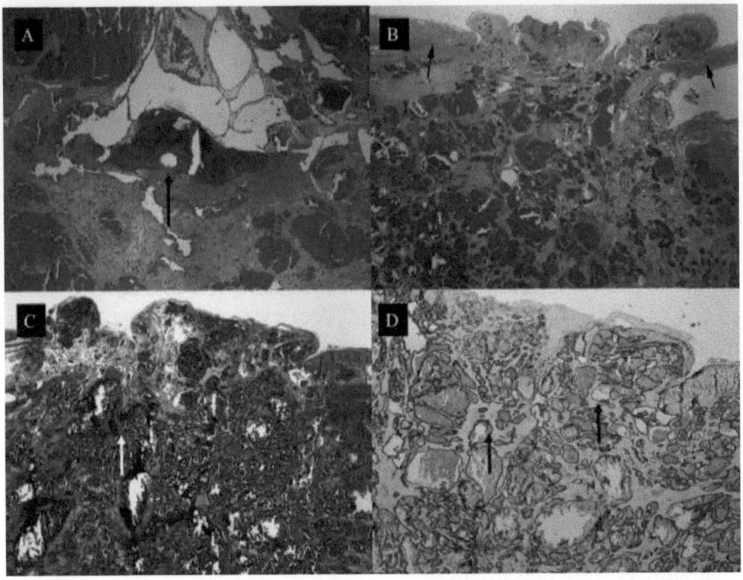

Figure 34(A) cavernous hemangioma: proliferation of small vessels with dilated lumen. H&E* × 100. (B) vessels infiltrate dura mater. H&E* × 100. (C) vessels separated by connective tissue. Picro Mallory ×100. (D) Immunohistochemistry with CD34 shows the boundaries of malformed vessels. ×100. *H&E: haematoxylin and eosin .[33].

Diagnosis can only be confirmed by histological study (Fig. 34), which shows highly dilated, thin-walled vessels with a venous component, surrounded by fibrous connective tissue [34]. The histological aspect of hemangiomacavernosa is identical regardless of the site where it develops (intra- or extraosseous) [34].

The diagnosis of hemangioma was confirmed in our patients by anatomopathological examination.

The natural evolution of the tumor is very slow, over several months or even years.

In our series, the time to consultation varied from 3 months to 4 years.

Therapeutically, the treatment of choice is en bloc resection of the tumor, combined with cranioplasty.

Radiotherapy is an alternative, stopping tumor progression without reducing tumor size, and is therefore reserved for inoperable tumors.

Curettage alone exposes the patient to the risk of local recurrence.

Finally, preoperative embolization can help prevent heavy bleeding in the case of large tumors.

Post-operative care is often straightforward, and no cases of recurrence at the surgical site have been reported [34].

In our series, all patients benefited from complete resection of the lesion, with simple postoperative care and a favorable outcome.

4. Histiocytosis X

4.1 Epidemiology

- Frequency :

It was first described by Jaffe and Lichtenstein in 1944; eosinophilic granuloma, together with Hand Schüller Christian disease and Letterer-Siwe disease, forms the histiocytosis X group.

It is rare, accounting for 7.5% of benign lesions with a tumoral appearance.

It accounts for 60% of cases of histiocytosis X [44,45].

- Location:

It can occur in all bones, but half of all sites are in the flat bones: the skull, pelvis and ribs.[46].

- Age/sex-ratio :

It almost exclusively affects children and young adults.
90% of patients were aged between 5 and 15 years, with a slight male predominance.[47,48].

4.2 Radiology

- STANDARD RADIOGRAPHY:

The granuloma typically takes the form of a rounded or oval, cookie-cutter lacuna, with more or less clear boundaries, depending on the stage of the disease, and varying in size from a few mm to a few cm. The confluence of several locations is responsible for a "map-like" appearance. It is intra-diploic, and secondarily destroys the external table or both external and internal tables. Non-symmetrical involvement of both tables is responsible for a bevelled or double-contour appearance. [47,44,46,49].

- CT :

It reveals a lacuna with either bevelled edges or a double contour, with a slightly hyperdense center in relation to the gray matter. The CT scan also reveals soft tissue mass. After injection of contrast medium, the central zone and periphery are contrasted, reflecting hypervascularization of the granulation tissue, while the rest of the lesion remains hypodense. CT is particularly advantageous for atypical forms, and allows better study of bone tables than radiophotographs[9,47,50].

- MRI:

The histiocytic lacuna is isosignal T1 and of heterogeneous signal in T2 weighting, after injection, gadolinium uptake is more marked at the periphery than in the center of the granuloma [8,47,51].

4.3. Histology

Together with "CHRISTIAN HAND SCHULLER" and "SIWE LETTERER" diseases, it forms the Langerhans cell histiocytosis or histiocytosis X group. At present, each disease is referred to by its extent, so we speak respectively of unifocal, multifocal or disseminated type cellular histiocytosis.

Pathogenesis is unknown, but generally considered to be inflammatory rather than tumoral.

The main cells show immunohistochemical and ultrastructural aspects of Langerhans cells[45,47,52,53].

- MACROSCOPY :

The lesion consists of mixed infiltration of Langerhans cells, chronic inflammatory cells including plasma cells and focal aggregates of eosinophils.

The presence of inflammatory cells within the cytoplasm of histiocytes is usually [47,48].

- IMMUNOHISTOCHEMISTRY :

Langerhans cells are clearly positive for S100 protein, vimentin and some histiocyte markers such as CD1a[48].

- ULTRASTRUCTURE :

the nuclear membrane is multilobulated, the appearance is that of a pentalaminar image with crossed striations and significant dilatation giving a "tennis racket" appearance[48].

4.4. Treatment

Treatment is surgical in the first instance.

Embolization is sometimes necessary prior to surgery, particularly in cases of invasion of the superior longitudinal sinus, as is often the case with giant cell tumors. This reduces intraoperative bleeding. It is performed via the trans-arterial route.[54,56,57,59].

There is no consensus on the management of HL in adults, and an extension work-up must be carried out.

Treatment indications depend on disease activity, the presence of high-risk sites (organs at risk, particular bone sites), and the possibility of local treatment.

In the case of bone involvement, spontaneous regression is possible. It can also be induced by curettage, or even a simple biopsy. In the case of pain, NSAIDs are often clearly effective, and may help the lesion to regress. Bone reconstruction is slow, rarely visible before 6 months. Extensive excisions run the risk of permanent loss of substance and should be avoided. Local corticosteroid injections may be suggested (methylprednisolone, 40 to 160 mg). Bone damage at risk is an indication for systemic treatment, based on a combination of vinblastine and corticosteroids. For rare aggressive forms, intensive polychemotherapy (MACOP-B, Special C) has also been reported.

In the future, new targeted therapies targeting the RAF-MEK-ERK pathway, such as vemurafenib, could enrich the therapeutic arsenal. [62].

5. Intraosseous meningioma

✧ **Intraosseous meningioma:** or "ectopic meningioma" is a generally benign tumor that can be found in the skin, facial sinuses and nasal cavities, orbits, neck and diploea of the cranial vault. In the skull, this lesion is always located in contact with a suture, usually coronal, or a fracture site[63,664].

The swelling is firm and tender, with infiltration of the integuments.

In the literature, only a few cases of cranial vault meningiomas are associated with intracranial hypertension, caused by intracranial thickening of the cranial vault with or without associated perifocal edema [63,64,65].

5.1. Epidemiology

- Frequency

Intraosseous meningiomas are rare, slow-growing tumors.

They represent less than 2% of all meningiomas[64].

- Location

The most frequently reported location of meningiomas is the frontotemporal region [65].

- Age/sex-ratio

Two frequency peaks were reported at the time of diagnosis, one in the second decade and another between the fifth and seventh decades.

Both sexes are almost equally affected [63].

5.2. Radiology

➤ Standard radiography:

It takes two forms:

The hyperostotic form, with thickening of the arch, sometimes bristling with spicules and "sunburst" bones.

The osteolytic or erosive form with bone lysis, with or without signs of reconstruction.

➤ CT :

- The hyperostotic form: this shows a stocky, regularly arranged appearance of spicules, unlike the fine, anarchic appearance of a malignant tumor.

- The osteolytic form: there are no particular signs[27,64].

➤ MRI:

It provides better anatomical definition, with marked hyposignal on T1- and T2-weighted sequences. Intravenous injection of gadolinium leads to contrast enhancement within the intraosseous component and in the meningeal envelopes opposite.

All authors describe the superiority of CT over MRI for the detection of lesions and the bony extension of the tumor[64, 777]

MRI combined with slow-flow magnetic resonance angiography (MRA) can be used to detect dural sinus invasion.

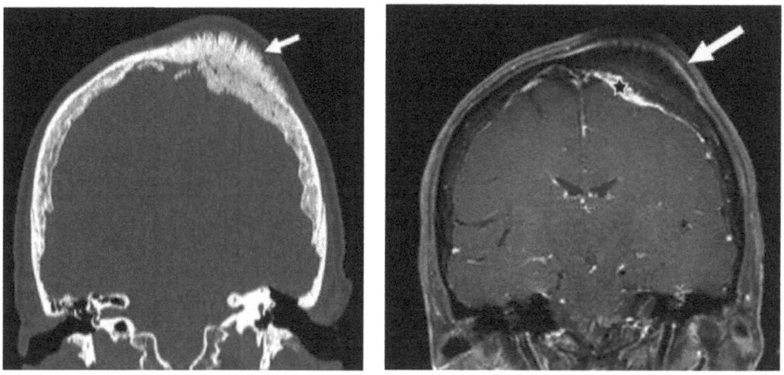

Figure 35Bone meningioma (A) Cerebral CT - coronal slice shows a hyperostatic lesion of the left parietal bone with peripheral speculation. (B)-MRI T1 coronal section after gadolinium injection: peripheral contrast with dural reaction. [40].

5.3. Histology

The pathogenesis of cranial vault meningiomas is controversial, three theories have been proposed:

AZARKIA et al hypothesized that a portion of the dura mater, containing arachnoid cells, is trapped in the line of the suture during embryonic development and subsequently gives rise to intraosseous meningiomas[65].

The second hypothesis is that the dural substance is enclosed in the fracture lines (if there is a history of trauma).

The third hypothesis was proposed by SHUANGSHOTI et al, who claimed that meninges are of mesenchymal origin, multipotential, can be divided into: fibrous, mucoid, adipose, synovial, cartilaginous, bone, hematopoietic, vascular and reticuloendothelial tissues. Meningiomas are caused by mesenchymal precursors in response to an as yet unidentified stimulus.[63,664].

- Macroscopy :

Most meningiomas are soft, with a smooth surface and dural attachment.

- Microscopy :

Fibrous lesions are firm and resistant in section; calcifications and ossifications are seen.

The diagnosis of certainty is based on histological examination. It is generally a benign tumor of the meningoendothelial or transitional type, rarely fibroblastic, angiomatous or psammomatous[64].

In 5 to 10% of cases, the meningioma is malignant, sarcomatous or anaplastic.

5.4 Differential diagnosis

This is mainly the case for osteolytic forms with metastases, osteosarcoma and myelomatous lacunae.

In the case of hyperostotic forms, the differential diagnosis is osteoma, fibrous dysplasia and Paget's disease.

5.5. Treatment

Surgical resection is only recommended when they are symptomatic. It remains the treatment of choice, combined with reconstruction of the bone defect.

Some authors recommend conventional radiotherapy for non-operable meningiomas or recurrences, but the results of radiotherapy remain debatable.[57,66-69].

In the case of intracranial meningiomas of frontal location, the operative tactics adopted are standardized as follows [61,63,70]:

Dorsal decubitus position, with 3-point headrest, placed as low as possible to perform a large bicornal scalp, which will free as much of the invaded epicranium as possible in the healthy zone; otherwise, it must be carefully preserved during scalping and flap trimming;the limits of the flap are easily identified visually and by palpation of the vault; a multitude of drill holes are made around the tumour, to create a wide bone trench of healthy bone. The dura is then rigorously suspended. The bone flap is then progressively lifted with a spatula and finger from all sides. Tumoral infiltration of the intracranial meningioma through the internal table of the bone reduces the risk of venous haemorrhage that would occur if the venous sinus were permeable. The intracranial time required is identical in every respect to that of a conventional para-sagittal meningioma. A compression bandage is applied to the scalp for several days at a time, to prevent constant effusions of cerebrospinal fluid due to resorption disorders; evacuating lumbar punctures are also performed during the first week.

B. Malignant tumors

1.osteosarcoma

1.1 Epidemiology

- Frequency :

Also known as osteogenic sarcoma, osteosarcoma is the second most common primary malignant bone tumour after myeloma, accounting for 40% of all cases.[71],[72].

It often affects the long bones, with only 2% affecting the cranial vault.[73].

JEFFERY et al reviewed 1,200 cases of osteosarcoma, 13 (1%) of which were located in the cranial vault.[72,74].

In our series, we encountered this tumor in a single case.

- Location:

The preferred site is the metaphysis of the long bones near the knee.[75].

In the cranial vault, the main site is the posterior convexity [74],[76]. It is generally a solitary lesion, but multiple involvement has been reported in 2% of cases[77].

- Age/sex-ratio :

Intraosseous meningioma occurs at a later age than in other localizations, generally in the 2ème -3ème decades with a female predominance and a sex ratio of 1 male to 1.9 females[72].

After the age of 40, osteosarcomas are either radiation-induced (after irradiation of a brain tumour), secondary to degeneration of Paget's disease, or developed on pre-existing fibrous dysplasia secondary to osteochondromatosis or chronic osteomyelitis. [72,74].

Osteosarcomas secondary to irradiation, Paget's disease or fibrous dysplasia occur in older patients and their incidence is estimated at 0.7 to 1% of cases in each of these three situations [73].

Cotton et al estimate that 5% of osteosarcomas are radiation-induced.[40]. Our case was a 23-year-old man, and we found no evidence of irradiation.

1.2 Radiology

- Standard radiography:

Radiological aspects are comparable to those of other localizations. In most cases, the lesion is osteolytic or mixed, with a mineralized matrix destroying the external and internal tables, causing irregular bone erosions, soft tissue invasion and, rarely, intracranial invasion. An anarchic periosteal reaction may be seen, manifested by bone spicules perpendicular to the cranial vault and codman spurs. Invasion of the scalp and dural plane is rapid and extensive, giving a "grass fire" appearance[10,71,74].

- CT :

It is superior to conventional images in the study of bone tables, reinforcing the probability of malignancy, while the presence of calcification provides topographical information and analyzes the brain parenchyma.

- MRI:

It provides better delineation of intramedullary and extraosseous extension, with a heterogeneous, predominantly intermediate signal on T1-weighted sequences and a T2 hypersignal. Gadolinium injection improves detection of small intra-diploid lesions.

CT and MRI are complementary: calcifications and bone remodeling are better analyzed by CT, while MRI more clearly visualizes associated vascular involvement and tumor extension within the diploea (disappearance of the physiological fatty hypersignal of the marrow, which is replaced by a tissue T1 hyposignal). Contrast is intense due to tumor hypervascularization.[72,53,27].

➤ ANGIOGRAPHY:

The tumor is hypervascular, with dilated pedicles and arteriovenous shunts, which can be demonstrated by standard MRI. In our series, the patient with osteosarcoma underwent a skull X-ray and a cerebral CT scan.

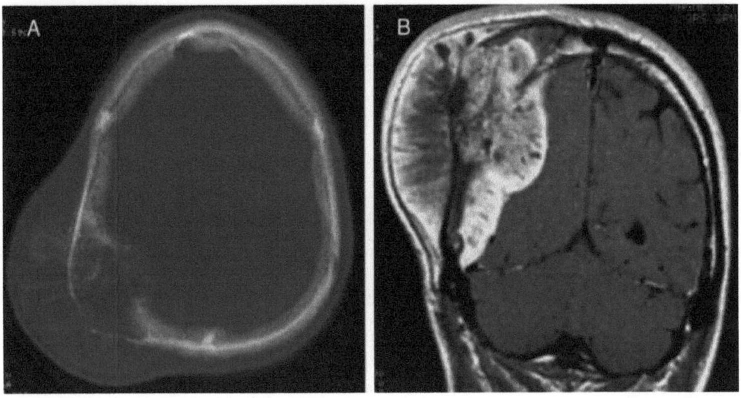

A) B)

Figure 36 Osteosarcoma. A. CT axial section bone window shows a large parietal osteolytic lesion with specules .B. T1 coronal section showing intense contrast uptake by the mass.[9].

1.3 Histology

Histologically, osteosarcomas are classified into three histological groups, according to the predominance of osteoblastic, chondroblastic and fibroblastic cells. [73].

The major criterion for positive diagnosis is the constant production of an osteoid matrix by tumour cells [73].

- Macroscopic

Osteosarcoma is a solid, hard, irregular tumor described as a fir tree on radiological examinations, due to tumoral spicules of calcified bone radiating at right angles[74,777].

- Microscopy :

Osteosarcoma is characterized by the presence of osteoid cells in the tumor. The tumor cells are highly pleomorphic (anaplastic), some of them giant, with numerous atypical mitoses. These cells produce osteoids describing irregular trabeculae (amorphous, eosinophilic) with or without central calcification[76].

1.4 differential diagnosis

The differential diagnosis is with chondrosarcoma and aggressive osteoblastoma. The appearance on imaging is the same, but there are some signs of aggressiveness, such as an unusual periosteal reaction. Epidemiological data (age, location on the bone) will help, but the final diagnosis is histological and biopsy is always essential[73].

1.5. Processing

Treatment involves neoadjuvant chemotherapy and surgery , osteosarcoma being not very radiosensitive [78].

Depending on the extent of locoregional extension and response to chemotherapy, surgical treatment is preferably conservative. It consists of wide surgical resection of the affected bone and invaded soft tissues, with bone reconstruction [40,78].

Today, chemotherapy has increased the survival rate of localized osteosarcomas to 70% at 3 years. This rate has remained stable over the last 20 years [79].

Multidrug therapy has also revolutionized the prognosis of osteosarcomas since its introduction in the various protocols. [80,81]. According to Maurizio Salvati et al. it should be used both neoadjuvantly and adjuvantly [69,72] . In this way, according to a prospective study [82]it would increase the two-year prognosis from 15-17% to 55-60%.

A retrospective study of 201 patients showed that the two-year survival curve of patients with craniofacial osteosarcoma, some of whom had been treated with complete surgical resection, was comparable to that of those whose surgery was incomplete but who received complementary polychemotherapy [83]. Obviously, the best survival rate in these cases is observed in patients who have undergone complete surgery combined with adjuvant chemotherapy.

Our patient underwent surgical excision of the tumor twice, with two courses of chemotherapy followed by adjuvant radiotherapy. He died after 5 months with local recurrence.

2. Chondrosarcoma

The clinical symptomatology of chondrosarcoma is not specific and depends on its location.

2.1. Epidemiology

- Frequency :

Chondrosarcoma accounts for 6% of all bone tumours and11% of primary malignant tumours.[84]It is the 1ère malignant tumor of the cartilaginous lineage and accounts for less than 1% of all intracranial tumors.[85]and it is much less rare in the cranial vault: less than 6% of vault tumors.

- Location:

It is mainly located on the temporal bone, especially in the petrous portion, followed by the spheno-occipital region, often due to an endochondral cartilage residue.

- Age/sex-ratio:

Male predominance is most often reported.

It generally occurs during the 4ème and 5ème decade.[77].

2.2. Radiology

- Standard radiography:

It shows geographic osteolysis and calcifications typical of cartilage tumours, which, when typical, are annular, arciform or "popcorn" shaped. Their abundance would be an argument in favour of chondroma, particularly if they occupy more than two-thirds of the lesion. Periosteal appositions may be absent or uninterrupted, benign in appearance, associated with cortical thickenings[79].

- CT :

Allows better assessment of: cortical lysis, periosteal appositions, tumor density close to that of cartilage (approximately 50 HU), anarchic intra-tumoral calcifications and intradural extension.[84].

➢ MRI:

Chondrosarcomas show heterogeneous contrast after gadolinium injection, with global T2-weighted hypersignal, hyposignal septa and calcifications. After gadolinium injection, the characteristic appearance of cartilage tumors is that of "arcs and rings" enhancement of the septa and periphery of the lesion.[86,87].

2.3 Histology

➢ Macroscopy :

Chondrosarcoma is a proliferation of malignant chondrocytes characterized by cyto-nuclear abnormalities within cartilage lobules, with no bone tissue formation.

➢ Microscopy :

Cytological and histological abnormalities usually classify chondrosarcomas into three grades of increasing malignancy[85,86].

- GRADE I: low malignancy; characterized by chondrocytic abnormalities (enlarged, binucleated nuclei), frequent calcifications.

- GRADE II: moderate malignancy; cytological abnormalities more frequent, calcifications rarer.

- GRADE III: high malignancy characterized by major chondrocytic abnormalities, mitoses and some degree of cellular anaplasia.

2.4. Differential diagnosis

The differential diagnosis is osteosarcoma and osteoblastomaagressif.

2.5. Processing

Treatment involves neoadjuvant chemotherapy and surgery.

II.Secondary tumors

A. Metastases

1. Epidemiology

- Frequency :

Metastases are the most frequent cause of cranial vault tumours in adults, with breast and lung cancers the most frequently implicated, followed by kidney and thyroid; prostate cancer, although osteophilic, has less affinity for the skull[88,89].

- **Osteolytic metastases**: breast cancer followed by lung cancer account for 80% of osteolytic metastases of the vault. 10% of metastases are single, most are multiple, and their number is underestimated as they only become visible when 50% of the bone structure has been destroyed[90,91].

- **Osteoblastic metastasis**: mostly seen in prostate, breast and bladder cancer, medulloblastoma and small-cell lung cancer.

Condensing metastases are much rarer than lytic forms, and are exceptional in the cranial vault.[92].

✧ **Mixed metastasis**: seen in breast, lung, prostate and neuroblastoma, but the cranial vault metastasis is almost always from breast cancer [93].

More than 60% of cancer patients have or develop bone metastases during the course of their cancer. [94].

They are rarely diagnosed clinically, and are frequently discovered in autopsies. [88].

In our series, we recorded 9 cases of metastasis, led by thyroid carcinoma (2 cases), breast (2 cases) followed by prostate cancer (1 case), one case of bronchial carcinoma and one locoregional metastasis.

- **Metastases extending to the cranial vault**

Invasion of the vault by contiguity from intra- or extra-cranial metastatic sites is possible. It is uncommon from the scalp, and mainly concerns malignant melanoma metastases.

Subdural and epidural metastases may extend to the cranial vault. These are mainly secondary to breast, lung and prostate cancer.[88].

In HEALY's series of 250 intracranial metastases, 7.6% invasions of the cranial vault were reported [90,95].

In 1889, Paget reported 36 cases of cranial metastases among 650 autopsies of patients with breast cancer.

Nagamine reported 12 cases (2.5%) of cranial metastases among 473 patients with thyroid cancer.

In 1981, Constant et al published the results of a study including 14 patients with cranial vault metastases. They found that in 42.85% of cases, the appearance of metastases preceded that of the primary tumour. [96].

Although they can cause severe disability through compression of dural sinuses or nerve structures, many metastatic skull lesions are asymptomatic. Spread by the hematogenous route, they represent the most frequent cause of skull vault tumors in adults. All cancers can metastasize to the skull vault. However, primary tumors of epithelial origin are the most frequent.

Table VII Summary of patient data from the study by M. Artico et al.

Patient no.	Age	Gender	Primary lesion	ASA classification	Location of secondary tumor	Number of hospital days	Suites
1	45	M	Prostate cancer	2	Vertex	4	6 months (deceased)
2	48	M	Melanoma	2	Occipital squama	5	2 years
3	58	M	Prostate cancer	2	Vertex	5	9 months (deceased)
4	58	F	Squamous cell lung cancer	2	Frontal bone	4	2 years
5	61	M	Adenocarcinoma of the lung	3	Left parietal bone	7	1 year (deceased)
6	63	F	Breast cancer	3	Occipital squama	8	4 years (deceased)
7	65	F	Breast cancer	3	Temporal and parietal bones (left)	10	3 years
8	66	M	Squamous cell lung cancer	3	Right occipital and parietal bones	12	6 months
9	68	M	Colon	3	Left parietal	5	1 year (decease

			cancer		bone		d)
10	70	M	Bladder cancer	2	Right parietal bone	5	6 months (decease d)

2. Radiology

➢ Standard radiology

The most common appearance is that of multiple rounded or oval lacunae, with no peripheral condensing reaction.[96].

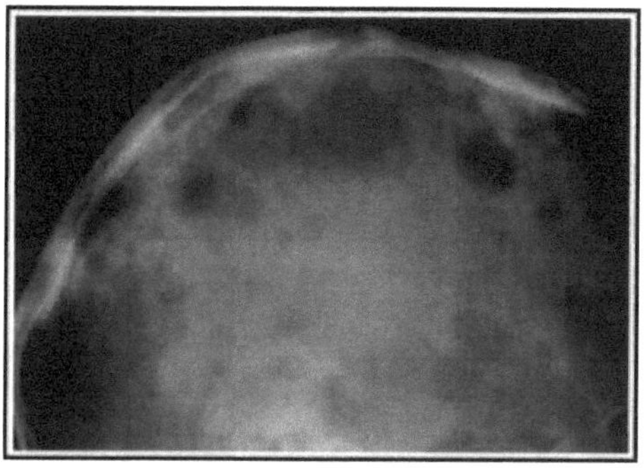

Figure 37 Metastasis of breast origin. Profile radiograph. Multiple lacunae without peripheral condensing reaction.

➢ CT SCAN

Lesions are usually osteolytic (lung, kidney, thyroid). The association of these with condensed areas, or even pure osteoblastic involvement, should prompt a search for prostatic or mammary origin. It is important to note that the same tumour may, in the same patient, give rise to osteolytic or osteosclerotic metastases (generally on different bones). Involvement is unique in only 10% of cases.[97].

They are initially located in the diploea, secondarily eroding the internal and external tables and finally extending into the soft tissue and extradural space.[40].

- MRI

In MRI, contrast injection is not necessary for the diagnosis of large metastases, but it does improve the detection of small intradiploid lesions. MRI also provides better information than CT on the degree of dural infiltration or invasion of a venous sinus. Lesions metastatic to the skull vault appear hypointense on T1 sequences, while hyperintense on T2; they generally show contrast enhancement on gadolinium injection, except those with a significant osteoblastic component. A periosteal reaction is rarely found[40,96].

3. Histology

In any case, the definitive diagnosis is histological, based on biopsy or tumour excision. For example, in 1889, Paget's disease, evoked in 36 out of 650 patients, turned out to be breast cancer after post-mortem examination[98].

4.differential diagnosis

The differential diagnosis of single foci of metastatic carcinomas to the vault is difficult, clinically and by conventional radiology, with primary bone tumors (solitary myeloma, osteogenic sarcoma, Ewing's sarcoma,) and even with non-tumoral lesions such as a focus of eosinophilic granuloma.

5. Treatment

From a technical point of view, cranial vault tumors are generally approached according to the principle of one-stage excision-reconstruction [99].

Surgical excision is recommended in the following circumstances: presence of a neurological deficit, massive bone destruction and/or dural infiltration, presence of a painful mass, presence of a solitary metastasis.

In the latter case, excision must remove the affected bone and adjacent skin tissue, whereas the dura must be preserved when it is macroscopically healthy.[100].

Surgical resection of cranial metastases always leaves a bone defect, which often requires reconstruction either with autogenous materials (such as broken ribs or iliac bone) or with alloplastic materials (calcium ceramics or polymers)[101].

According to several authors, surgical resection cannot influence the underlying disease, but it does enable the patient to avoid pain and local discomfort. It may also improve neurological symptoms[102].

External radiotherapy may be indicated in the case of inoperable metastases and in the presence of tumour excision margins[67].

In the literature, survival of patients with cranial vault metastases varies between 14 months and 4.5 years [100].

Neoadjuvant and adjuvant chemotherapy are reputed to eradicate micro-metastases and necrotize the tumour and its vascular ramifications, thus enabling more conservative surgery. [74] Chemotherapy has also been shown to reduce the risk of local relapse and the number of metastases, as well as lengthening the time required for their formation.

Table VIII Epidemiology of some arch lesions

		Histological type	Frequency	Gender	Age (years)	Common locations
Primary tumors	**Benign tumors**	Epidermoid cyst	0.6% of cranial vault tumors		20-60	Parietal frontal bone
		Osteoma	20% of primary vault tumors		40-50	Frontal sinus ethmoidal sphenoidal bone
		Osteoblastoma	1% of all bone tumors	M	20-30	Temporal bone
		Hemangioma	10% of benign bone tumors of the vault	F	40-50	Parietal bone Frontal bone
		Aneurysmal bone cyst	2.5% of primary bone tumours	F	Young adult	Parietal bone
		Chondroma osteochondroma	0.16% of cranial tumors			Frontoparietal bone

		Giant cell tumor	9% of benign primary bone tumors	F	20-30	Sphenotemporal bone
		Eosinophilic granuloma	Rare		Child + young adult	
		Chordoma	Exceptional	M	30-40	Occipital bone
		Myxoma	Rare	-	20-30	Parieto-temporal bone
		Ossifying fibroma	Rare			
		Hydatidosis	Rare			
		Lipoma	0.1% of all bone tumors			Frontal bone Parietal bone
		Chondroblastoma	1% of all bone tumors	M	10-20	Temporal bone
	Malignant tumors	Osteosarcoma	40% of primary malignant tumors	F	20-30	Occipital bone

		Ewing's sarcoma	0.6% of malignant bone tumors		10-25	Frontal bone Parietal bone
		Chondrosarcoma	Rare		50	Parietal bone
		Fibrosarcoma	10% of primary malignant bone tumors	-	30-60	
Secondary tumors	**Hematogenic**	Multiple myeloma	The most common primary bone tumor	M	50-60	
		Solitary plasmacytoma	2.5% of primary bone tumours		< 50	Parietal frontal occipital bone
		LMNH	3.4% of primary bone tumours	F	30-40	Parietal frontal-occipital bone
		LMH	Rare	F	30-40	Parietal frontal-occipital bone

	Metastases	Metastases	The most common tumor of the vault			
	Neighborhood tumor extending to the vault	Meningioma	50% at VC level			Coronal suture
		Extensive metastasis to the VC	Uncommon			
		Scalp tumor	Rare			External table/diploë

Table IXEpidemiology of some skull vault tumors according to sex, age, tumor site and frequency.

Tumors	**Gende r**	**Preferred age**	**Preferential tumor site**	**Frequency**
Squamous cell cyst[3]	Indiffe rent [5]	20-60 years [11]	Neighbouring pterion + lateral parts of coronal suture, fronto-parietal	0.2% to 1% of cranial tumors according to Pertuiset, Russel DS et al.
Osteoma[19]	♀= ♂	40 - 50 years	Parietal	1 %
Osteosarcoma[72]		10 - 25 years	Posterior convexity	0,7 à 3%
Hemangioma[39]	♀>♂	40 - 50 years	Parietofrontal	1% of primary bone tumors
Ewing's sarcoma[103]		10-25 years	Frontal and parietal convexities	Rare

Table X (Continued): Distribution of some skull vault tumors according to sex, age, tumor site and frequency.

Tumors	**Gender**	**Age of preferenc e**	**Preferential tumor site**	**Frequency**
Kahler's disease[104]	♂+++	50-60 years old	Disseminated in the vault	Rare
Solitary plasmacytoma[105]	♂=♀	< 50 years	Occipital and parietal	0,7%
Meningiomas [61]	♀+++	50-60 years	Large wing of the sphenoid	
Fibrous dysplasia[106]	♀ = ♂	0 - 30 years	Fronto-orbital	

Paget's disease[107]	♂>♀	>50 years	Scattered	25 - 65% of myeloma cases [108]

♀ = woman   ♂ = male   < = inferior>   = superior

CONCLUSION

Tumor localization in the cranial vault is rare. Data in the literature concerning the frequency of bone tumours and the cranial location of primary tumours vary from 0.8% to 2%. [109]. Tumors of the skull vault are essentially dominated by secondary lesions.

Tumors of the skull vault affect both children and adults. In children and adolescents, they are dominated by epidermoid and dermoid cysts. [35]. They are also secondary to neuroblastoma metastases. In adolescents, they are most often osteomas. In adults, on the other hand, the origin is more diverse, and dominated by breast and lung cancer metastases [40,90,110].

None of the authors of the articles we found emphasized a particular gender predominance. Gender predominance is a function of the tumour itself. Some tumors, such as meningioma or hemangioma, are more likely to be found in women, while others, such as Kahler's disease or Paget's disease, predominate in men.

We found no elective site on the skull vault for tumor localization. Tumor location varies according to the tumor involved. Metastases, the most common tumors in the vault, are generally multiple. Primary tumors, such as epidermoid cysts, have a preferential frontal, parietal or occipital location.

Apart from the embryological origin of certain tumors, others are favored by trauma or radiotherapy. Genetic origin is also sometimes found.

We report a retrospective study about 20 cases of cranial vault tumors, managed at the Neurosurgery Department of the Main Military Hospital of Instruction in Tunis over a 17-year period from January 1, 2000 to December 31, 2016.

The aim of this work is to study the epidemiological, clinical, radiological and therapeutic aspects of cranial vault tumors in our series, and to assess the short- and long-term evolution and prognosis.

The overall study of the 20 patients revealed the following results:

1. Epidemiological :

The mean age of our patients was 47.4 years, with extremes ranging from 20 to 75 years. The majority were between 40 and 50 years of age.

The gender breakdown showed a slight male predominance, with a sex ratio of 1.2.

2. Clinically:

The most frequent reason for consultation was the finding of swelling in 9 cases, associated in 8 cases with headaches.

Discovery was fortuitous in three cases.

For our patients, the time to consultation ranged from 4 months to 12 years.

Clinical examination revealed :

Swelling lasted in 8 cases, firm in one.

No neurological deficit was found on initial examination.

3. Paraclinical :

Skull X-rays were performed in 7 patients, showing bone lysis in 6 and osteocondensation in 1.

CT scans were performed on our20 patients, and allowed us to :

a) Locate lesions on :

- Frontal bone in 8 cases.
- Parietal bone in 7 cases.
- Temporal bone in 1 case.
- Occipital bone in 4 cases.

Multiple localization was found in 2 cases.

The location was essentially frontal and parietal.

b) Determining lesion size: more than half were between 2 and 4cm in size.

c) Determination of lesion density: lesions were hyperdense in 7 cases, hypodense in 10 and mixed in 3.

Cerebral MRI was performed in 4 patients, in addition to CT in 3 cases, and immediately in 1 case, enabling identification and evaluation of the tissue component, and localization of the tumor and its relationships.

Bone scintigraphy was performed in 4 patients as part of the extension workup, showing a single skull lesion in 2 cases.

4. Therapeutically:

Complete excision was performed in 16 patients, and subtotal excision in 3. Cranioplasty was performed in 19 cases.

Four patients underwent postoperative radiotherapy and adjuvant chemotherapy.

Patients with secondary localization were referred to a medical oncologist for follow-up therapy.

Therapeutic abstention was indicated in a case of cranial vault metastasis, in a woman in poor general condition with metastases in other locations.

5. Histologically:

We found 11 cases of benign lesions: 4 osteomas, 2 cashemangiomas, 2 cases of histiocytosis X, 1 case of neurofibroma, 1 case of intraosseous meningioma and 1 case of epidermoid cyst.

Malignant tumors were diagnosed in 2 cases. These were an osteosarcoma and a chondrosarcoma.

Secondary lesions were found in 9 cases.

6. On an evolutionary level:

Immediate evolution was favorable in the majority of cases.

After a mean follow-up of 12 months, with extremes ranging from 4 months to 15 years, the posterior outcome was favorable in 60% of cases, with no recurrence.

One patient was lost to follow-up and two patients died.

Prognosis depended essentially on the histological nature of the tumour. The prognosis was favorable in all cases of benign tumors, and unfavorable in 11 cases: 2 cases of primary malignant tumors, 9 cases of secondary lesions.

Overall, our results are in line with those reported in the literature.

In conclusion: Cranial vault tumors are a rare entity,

The revealing clinical symptom is often a cranial swelling.

Etiological diagnosis is based on a comparison of clinical, radiological and anatomopathological data.

A multitude of radiological and etiological differential diagnoses

The right practitioner can turn the prognosis around.

Treatment is often surgical, and in the case of malignant lesions, may be combined with radiotherapy and/or chemotherapy.

The key to proper management of vault tumors is knowledge of their histological type, on which the course and prognosis depend.

The limits of our work

One difficulty we encountered in data collection was that the files did not provide satisfactory information on the clinical and evolutionary status of our patients.

Given the small number of patients, we were unable to draw up statistical results.

The difficulty we encountered is linked to the paucity of publications on this subject. This in turn is linked to the rarity of tumors localized to the skull vault.

APPENDICES

APPENDIX 1: Vault tumor data entry form

I-Identification :
-Full name :
-Gender :
-Age :
-ATCD :
II-Clinical :
-Discovery mode :
-Consultation period :
-General review:
-Neurological examination :
-Examination of swelling:
□□Siège :
□□Taille :
□□Caractère painful :
□□Consistance :
□□Etat facing skin
III- Radiological examinations :
Skull X-ray:
-Cerebral CT :
-Brain MRI:
-bone scan :
-Other tests :
IV-Biology :
V-Processing :
-Medical :
-Surgical :
-Operative sequences :
-Radiotherapy :
-Chemotherapy
VI-Anatomopathological examination :
VII- Short- and long-term trends :

Appendix 2: Histological classification of cranial vault tumors

1. Osteogenic tumors s

1.1. Benign

-osteoma

- osteoid osteoma

- benign osteoblastoma

- exostosis

- ossifying fibroma

1.2 Malignant

-osteosarcoma

- paraosteal sarcoma

- periosteal sarcoma

- multicentric sarcoma

- telangiectatic sarcoma

- soft tissue sarcoma

2. Cartilage tumours

2.1. Benign

- chondroma

- osteochondroma

- chondroblastoma
- juxta-cortical chondroma
- chondromyxoid fibroma

2.2 Malignant

- chondrosarcoma

3. Giant cell tumors

4. Vascular tumors

4.1. Benign

- hemangioma
- lymphangioma
- cystic angiomatosis
- massive osteolysis
- glomus tumor
- hemangiopericytoma

4.2 Malignant

- hemangiosarcoma
- lymphangiosarcoma

5. Connective tissue tumors

5.1. Benign

- lipoma
- fibroma

5.2. Malignant

- liposarcoma
- fibrosarcoma

6. Other tumors

- chordoma
- neurofibroma
- meningioma
- chemodectoma
- leiomyoma and leiomyosarcoma
- squamous cell cyst

7. Hematological disorders

- Ewing's sarcoma
- Parker Jackson sarcoma
- lymphoma
- plasmacytoma, multiple myeloma
- leukemia
- ARAN chloroma or green cancer

8. Pseudotumors

- eosinophilic granuloma
- non-ossifying fibroma

- solitary bone cyst
- aneurysmal cyst
- brown hyperparathyroid tumors
- myositis ossificans

Giant cell tumors have their own specific architectural and evolutionary characteristics, making it difficult to regard them unreservedly as benign.

BIBLIOGRAPHICAL REFERENCES

1. Krupp W, Heckert A, Holland H, Meixensberger J, Fritzsch D. Giant intradiploic epidermoid cyst with large osteolytic lesions of the skull: a case report. J Med Case Rep. 2012;6(1):85.
2. Duan Z xin, Chu S hua, Ma Y bin, Zhang H, Zhu J liang. Giant intradiploic epidermoid cyst of the occipital bone. J Clin Neurosci. 2009;16(11):1478- 80.
3. Gaivas S, Rotariu D, Dumitrescu G, Iliescu B, Apetrei C, Poeata I. Intradiploic epidermoid cyst of the skull. Case report. Journal of Diagnostic Pathology 2014 ;9(2) :38.
4. Samdani S, Kalra GS, Rawat DS. Posttraumatic intradiploic epidermoid cyst of frontal bone. J CraniofacSurg. 2013;24(2):e128-2.
5. Yanai Y, Tsuji R, Ohmori S, Tatara N, Kubota S, Nagashima C. Malignant change in an intradiploic epidermoid: report of a case and review of the literature. Neurosurgery. 1985 Feb-cited 2017 ;16(2):252-6.
6. Özgi ray E, Perumal K, Çinar C, Emre K, Ertan Y, et al. Management of Calvarial Tumors: A Retrospective Analysis and Literature Review. Turk Neurosurg. 2016;(1).
7. Parlier-Cuau C, Brouard R, Laouisset L, Touraine S, Hamzé B, Petrover D, et al. Diagnosis of a cranial vault lacuna.Revue du Rhumatisme Monographs. 2013;80: 44-57.
8. Colas L, Caron S, Cotten A. Skull vault lesions: A review. American Journal of Roentgenology. 2015; 840-7.
9. O. Naggara, A. Goncalves, É. Meary,R. Souillard-Scemama , J.-F. Meder et al. Cranial vault tumors.radiology and medical imaging.2011;19.
10. Yalçin O, Yildirim T, Kizilkiliç O, Hürcan CE, Koç Z, Aydin V, et al. CT and MRI findings in calvarial non-infectious lesions. DiagnIntervRadiol .2007;13(2):68–74.
11. Hong B, Hermann EJ, Klein R, Krauss JK, Nakamura M. Surgical resection of osteolytic calvarial lesions: Clinicopathological features. Clin Neurol Neurosurg. 2010;112(10):865-9.
12. Bauduer F, Bessou M, Guyomarc'h P, Mercier C, Castex D. Multiple Calvarial Lytic Lesions: A Differential Diagnosis from Early Medieval France (5th to 7th c. AD). Int J Osteoarchaeol. 2014;24(5):665-74.
13. Amaral L, Chiurciu M, Almeida JR, Ferreira NF, Mendonça R, Lima SS. MR imaging for evaluation of lesions of the cranial vault: A pictorial essay. ArqNeuropsiquiatr. 2003;61:521–32.
14. Tucker WS, Nasser-Sharif FJ. Benign skull lesions Can J Surg. 1997;40(6):449-55.
15. Younghee Y, Won-Jin M, Hyeong S , Joon Cho, Myung HR.Pictorial Essay. J Korean Soc Radiol2016;74:43-54.
16. Lloret I, Server A, Taksdal I. Calvarial lesions: a radiological approach to diagnosis. Acta Radiol. 2009;50:531-42.

17. Binit S, Mittal M, Mittal A, Thukral B. Atypical lytic lesions of skull: Clinical and radiological correlation. Annals of Indian Academy of Neurology. 2014;50:52-59.
18. Xiao G. Giant hyperdense intradiploic epidermoid cyst of the skull with extra and intracranial extension: Report of two cases and literatures review. Chinese J Cancer Res. 2005;17(2):154-6.
19. Locatelli M, Alimehmeti R, Rampini P, Prada F. Intradiploic frontal epidermoid cyst in a patient with repeated head injuries: Is there a causative relationship. Acta Neurochir (Wien). 2006;148(10):1107–10.
20. Lee D-H. Intradiploic epidermoid cyst of the temporal bone: is it the same as or different from cholesteatoma. J Craniofac Surg. 2011;22(5):1973-5.
21. Constans JP, Meder JF, De Divitiis E, Donzelli R, Maiuri F. Giant intradiploic epidermoid cysts of the skull. J Neurosurg. 1985 ;8;62(3):445- 8.
22. K. Jaiswal, A. K. Mahapatra A. Giant intradiploic epidermoid cysts of the skull. A report of eight cases. Br J Neurosurg. 2000;14(3):225-8.
23. Ajja A, Akhaddar A, Naama O, Guazzaz M, Belhachmi A, AsriAbad C, et al. Intradiploid epidermoid cyst of the occipital bone. Neurosurgery. 2007;53(5):367-70.
24. Hasturk AE, Basmaci M, Yilmaz ER, Kertmen H, Gurer B, Atilgan AO. Giant intradiploic epidermoid cyst presenting as solitary skull mass with intracranial extension. J CraniofacSurg. 2013;24(6):2169-71.
25. Kano T, Ikota H, Kobayashi S, Iwasa S, Kurosaki S, Wada H. Malignant Transformation of an Intracranial Large Epidermoid Cyst With Leptomeningeal CarcinomatosisCase Report. Neurol Med Chir Malig. 2010;50(50):349-53.
26. Vellutini EAS, de Oliveira MF, Ribeiro APC, Rotta JM. Malignant transformation of intracranialepidermoidcyst. Br J Neurosurg. 2014;28(4):507-9.
27. Mitra I, Duraiswamy M, Benning J, Joy HM. Imaging of focal calvarial lesions. Vol. 71, Clinical Radiology. 2016; 389-98.
28. Deacu C-M, Iordan A, Baz R. Imaging evaluation of diffuse abnormalities of the cranial vault (Case report). ARS Medica Tomitana. 2015;21(2):95- 100.
29. Haddad FS, Haddad GF, Zaatari G. Cranial osteomas: their classification and management. Report on a giant osteoma and review of the literature. SurgNeurol. 1997;48(2):143-7.
30. Patel TR, Borah GL. Frontal bone periosteal osteomas. PlastReconstr Surg. 2004;114(3):648-51.
31. Ahmadi MS, Ahmadi M, Dehghan A. Osteoid osteoma presenting as a painful solitary skull lesion: a case report. Iran J Otorhinolaryngol. 2014 ;26(75):115-8.
32. J. Ognard,C.Barberot,M. Garetier,F. Abed Ra.Diagnosis of cranial osteocondensations and hyperostoses.2016:40:58-65
33. VISHWAKARMA R, Joseph ST, Patel KB, Sharma A. Giant frontal osteoma: case report with review of literature. Indian J Otolaryngol Head Neck Surg. 2011 ;63(Suppl 1):122-6.

34. Fan KL, Ghadjar K, Yuan JT, Lazaref J, Wilson L, Bradley JP. Giant Cranial Osteoma. J Craniofac Surg. 2012;23(5):480-2.
35. Dispenza C, Martines F, Dispenza F, Caramanna C, Saraniti C. Frontal sinus osteoma complicated by palpebral abscess: case report. Acta Otorhinolaryngol Ital. 2004;24(6):357-60.
36. Kang SH, Park SW, Kwon KY, Hong WJ. A solitary skull lesion of syphilitic osteomyelitis. J KoreanNeurosurg Soc. 2010;48(1):85-7.
37. Reale G, Ungari C, Riccardi E, Calvani F, Quarato D, Rinna C, et al. Fronto-ethmoidal osteoma. Open treatment. Ann Ital Chir. 2014;85(3):214-8.
38. Atesok KI, Alman B a., Schemitsch EH, Peyser A, Mankin HJ. Osteoid osteoma and osteoblastoma. J AcadOrthop Surg. 2011;19:678-89.
39. Couturier A, Aumaître O, Mom T, Gilain L, André M. La dysplasie fibreuse osseuse cranio-faciale.Revue de Medecine Interne. 2016;36:834-9.
40. Salunke P, Sinha R, Khandelwal NK, Kumar A, Gupta K, et al. Primary intraosseus cavernous hemangioma of the skull base. Br J Neurosurg. 2010;24(1):84-5.
41. Xu P, Lan S, Liang Y, Xiao Q. Multiple cavernous hemangiomas of the skull with dural tail sign: a case report and literature review. BMC Neurol 2013;13:155.
42. Yang Y, Guan J, Ma W, Li Y, Xing B, Ren Z, et al. Primary Intraosseous Cavernous Hemangioma in the Skull. Medicine (Baltimore). 2016;95(11):e3069.
43. Nasi D, Somma L di, Iacoangeli M, Liverotti V, Zizzi A, Dobran M, et al. Calvarial bone cavernous hemangioma with intradural invasion: An unusual aggressive course-Case report and literature review. Int J Surg Case Rep. 2016;22:79-82.
44. Park BH, Hwang E, Kim CH. Primary intraosseous hemangioma in the frontal bone. Archives of Plastic Surgery. 2013;40:283-5.
45. Dubbeldam A, Thywissen C, Vanwyck R, Cleeren P. Intraosseous hemangioma of the left parietal bone. JBR-BTR. 2015;98(3):117-8.
46. Atci IB, Albayrak S, Yilmaz N, Uçler N, Durdağ E, Ayden O, et al. Cavernous hemangioma of the parietal bone. Am J Case Rep. 2013;14:401- 4.
47. Heckl S, Aschoff A, Kunze S. Cavernomas of the skull: review of the literature 1975-2000. Neurosurg Rev. 2002;25(1-2):56-62-7.
48. Kirmani A, Sarmast A, Bhat A. A unique case of calvarial hemangioma. Surg Neurol Int. 2016;7(15):398.
49. Néel a, M. Artifoni , J. Donadieuc, G. Lorillonb, M. Hamidoua, A. Tazi b,d, et al.Histiocytoselangerhansienne de l'adulte Langerhans cellhistiocytosis in adults. Rev Med interne 2015;69(5):100-10.
50. Sauerborn D, Pajić-Penavić I, Stojadinović T. Eosinophilic granuloma of the temporal bone in an adult: controversies in the management. Coll Antropol. 2012;36:163-6.
51. Jin Lim S, Kwan Lim M, Won Park S, Eun Kim J, Hye Kim J, et al. Langerhans Cell Histiocytosis in the Skull: Comparison of MR Image and Other Images; J Korean Soc Magn Reson Med, 2014;13(1):74-80.

52. Davidson L, McComb JG, Bowen I, Krieger M. Craniospinal Langerhans cell histiocytosis in children: 30 years' experience at a single institution. J NeurosurgPediatr. 2008;1(3):187-95.
53. A case of calvarial eosinophilic granuloma with rapid expansion and wide skull invasion: immunohistochemical analysis of Ki-67. J Clin Neurosci. 2002;9(1):72-6.
54. Berhouma M, Krichen W, Chamseddine A, Jemel H. Surgical treatment of solitary eosinophilic granulomas of the skull vault. About two cases. Neurosurgery. 2009;55(6):555-9.
55. Multifocal bone langerhansian histiocytosis: place of radiotherapy.J Cancer Radiotherapy. 2010;14(8):759-62.
56. Henon A, Colombat M, Rodallec M, Redondo A, Feydy A. Intraosseous meningioma of the cranial vault: anatomo-radiological confrontation. J Radiol. 2005;86(1):83-5.
57. Yun JH, Lee SK. Primary osteolytic intraosseous atypical meningioma with soft tissue and dural invasion: Report of a case and review of literatures. J Korean Neurosurg Soc. 2014;56(6):509-12.
58. Kaptan h, Karaba P, Birler U, Köke F ,Kasamcan O et al.Intraosseous meningioma: Case report. TurkiyeKlinikleri Journal of Medical Sciences. 2011; 1736-9.
59. Choi KW, Chung KJ, Kim Y-H. Primary intraosseous meningioma. Arch Plast Surg. 2015;42(3):378-80.
60. Chen TC. Primary Intraosseous Meningioma. Neurosurgery Clinics of North America. 2016;32:189-93.
61. Caruso R, Fini G, Pesce A, Wierzbicki V, Marrocco L, Piccione E, et al. A primary intraosseous cystic meningioma: Case report. Int J Surg Case Rep. 2017;37:189-92.
62. Suri V, Singh A, Das R, Das A, Malhotra P, Jain S, et al. Osseous sarcoid with lytic lesions in skull. Rheumatol Int. 2014;34(4):579-82.
63. Mascarenhas L, Peteiro A, Ribeiro CA, Magalhaées Z, Româo H, Magalhaées F, et al. Skullosteosarcoma:illustratedreview. Acta Neurochir (Wien). 2004;146(11):1235-9.
64. Jroundi L, Barkouchi F, Chakir N, El Quessar A, Jiddane M, Bacadi D. Occipital osteosarcoma in a 33-year-old man: About a case report. J Radiol. 2006;87(1):62-4.
65. Salvati M, Ciappetta P, Raco A. Osteosarcomas of the skull. Clinical remarks on 19 cases. Cancer. 1993;71(7):2210-6.
66. Cho H, Park B-J, Park Y-K. Multifocal osteosarcoma of the skull: multiple primary or metastatic A case report. Korean J Pathol. 2014;48(2):146-50.
67. hadeleyc.,B.S.,loyola V. Gressot,AkashJ and al. osteosarcoma of the cranial vault and skull base in pediatric patients. J NeurosurgPediatr. 2014;13(13):380-7.
68. Smeele LE, Kostense PJ, van der Waal I, Snow GB. Effect of chemotherapy on survival of craniofacial osteosarcoma: a systematic review of 201 patients. J Clin Oncol. 1997;15(1):363-7.

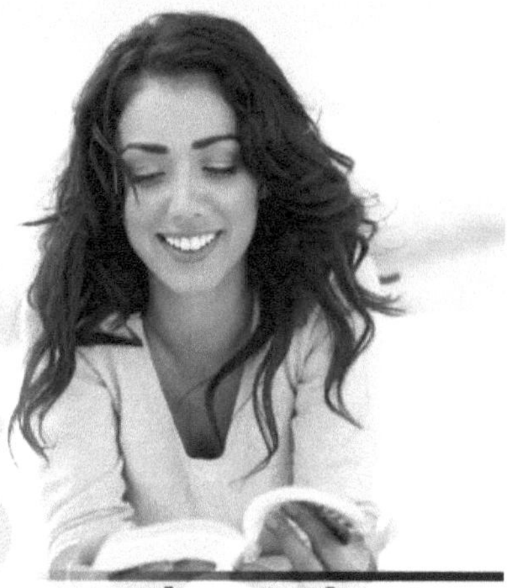

MIX
Papier aus verantwortungsvollen Quellen
Paper from responsible sources
FSC® C105338

Printed by Books on Demand GmbH, Norderstedt / Germany